ETHICS
for Everyone

A Practical Guide to Interdisciplinary Biomedical Ethics Education

Linda C. Grafius, Ed.D.

American Society for Healthcare Education and Training

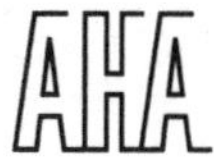

AHA books are published by American Hospital Publishing, Inc., an American Hospital Association company

Library of Congress Cataloging-in-Publication Data

Grafius, Linda C.
Ethics for everyone : a practical guide to interdisciplinary biomedical ethics education / Linda C. Grafius.
p. cm.
Includes bibliographical references.
ISBN 1-55648-134-9
1. Medical ethics—Study and teaching. 2. Bioethics—Study and teaching. I. Title.
R724.G764 1995
174'.2'071—dc20 95-3469
CIP

Catalog no. 058301

Printed in the USA

AHA is a service mark of the American Hospital Association used under license by American Hospital Publishing, Inc.

Text set in Goudy
3M—4/95—0405

Richard Hill, Senior Editor
Anne Hermann, Editor
Peggy DuMais, Production Coordinator
Luke Smith, Cover Designer
Marcia Bottoms, Books Division Executive Editor
Brian Schenk, Books Division Director

Dedicated, with love, to

My father,
and to
Rich,
Rebecca,
and
Benjamin

and to the memory of
Julia,
Frank,
and
Jean

Contents

List of Figures

About the Author

Linda C. Grafius, Ed.D, has worked in the fields of health care, education, and biomedical ethics for many years. She served as the administrative director of educational services at St. Mary Medical Center, Langhorne, Pennsylvania, where she was responsible for overseeing in-service and nursing education, community programs, cardiopulmonary resuscitation and first-aid courses, continuing medical education for physicians, the speakers' bureau, and audiovisual and media services. Dr. Grafius serves on the medical center's ethics committee and, in 1991, was instrumental in the development and implementation of an ethics grand rounds program. The St. Mary Medical Center model for grand rounds was subsequently adopted by several other hospitals in the Franciscan Health System.

Before joining the staff at St. Mary Medical Center, Dr. Grafius was patient and guest relations coordinator at Doylestown Hospital in Doylestown, Pennsylvania, and director of mental retardation services and coordinator of hospice and bereavement counseling services at the Lenape Valley Foundation, which is also located in Doylestown.

Dr. Grafius received her doctorate in health education from Temple University in Philadelphia, where she was awarded the Sarah Leeds Miller Doctoral Award for outstanding scholarship and service in university and community activities. She has served on the local board of directors for the American Heart Association and the Special Olympics and is a past president of the Southeastern Pennsylvania chapter of the American Society for Healthcare Education and Training (ASHET).

Preface

Soon the splendor of the setting sun will slip down behind the hills. The wavering path of gold across the lake will fade. Sky and water will be painted with scarlet, orange and pink, deepening to a dusky purple, sapphire, then smoky gray. We have seen many such sunsets. Never two alike, but always stealing like a benediction into our consciousness to remind us that ours is a good and beautiful world.

Kate Smith
Lake Placid, NY
August 25, 1938

The world in which we live is indeed a good and beautiful place. One of the elements that makes it so is the broad and complex diversity of the people who inhabit it. However, that very diversity—the way we do things and the reasons why we do them—at times can create situations in which conflicts and dilemmas develop. Such conflicts can be particularly difficult when they involve issues related to terminal and chronic illness or death and dying. What is right or ethical for one individual may seem very wrong or unethical to another.

In their jobs, health care workers are frequently called on to help sort out ethical issues so that patients and family can make decisions in the best interests of themselves and their loved ones. Providing such assistance is not an easy task, and health care workers may find it troublesome to be asked to do so. In some cases, a situation may not be handled in the best possible manner, not because the health care worker has not attempted to do so, but because he or she has not been given the appropriate training and the resources that are needed to know *what* to do and *how* to do it.

Over the years, I have been involved in a number of cases in which the handling of a situation with a patient or a patient's family has troubled me—cases when things could have or should have been done differently; cases when communication broke down, or people felt uncomfortable dealing with difficult circumstances. Sometimes conflicts arose and no one was available to help resolve them, or patients and families simply did not understand what was happening with their care.

Julia's was one such case. She had frequently expressed a desire to die, and her family faced an ethical dilemma as her condition deteriorated. At age 102 she was blind, bedridden, and in chronic pain from arthritis. Julia was completely lucid and deeply religious. Her main topic of conversation was her readiness to "go home to the Lord," where she believed she would be reunited with her husband and sons who had preceded her in death decades ago. When Julia had a stroke and lost her ability to swallow, her grandchildren were asked if they wanted her to have a feeding tube inserted. After much discussion that centered on her loving family's desire not to contribute to her death, a tube was inserted, and the end of Julia's life was delayed.

Another case involved Frank, a 47-year-old former army officer who was divorced and lived alone. He had diabetes and had been blind for several years. Physicians had recently recommended the amputation of his gangrenous feet. Although his condition continued to deteriorate, Frank refused most treatment and did not take his insulin on a regular basis. According to his sister, Frank was frequently depressed, but he received no psychological or psychiatric assessments and interventions. The day before Christmas, Frank was found dead in bed. He had been dead for more than a week.

A third case concerned Jean, who had cirrhosis of the liver that was the result of chronic hepatitis of unknown origin. Her husband and daughter had frequently asked Jean's physician about her treatment options and her prognosis. Jean and her family were assured that everything was being done and that she would be able to go home shortly. They were told that she would be able to live a full and healthy life. However, Jean never left the hospital. The day before she died, Jean's husband was called and told "to get to the hospital immediately because she won't last the day." As her family sat with her for the next 28 hours, no physician visited or even called. The last thing Jean said before lapsing into her final coma was, "I'm afraid."

The three cases just described provide examples of unaddressed and unresolved issues: issues that could be called ethical dilemmas. These examples are not unusual cases. They are typical of the types of situations that health care workers, patients, and families face every day as they attempt to cope with chronic or terminal illness and with death.

These particular cases were more troubling to me than most ethical dilemmas, because I personally lived through them. Julia was my adopted "grandmother," Frank was a dear friend from my undergraduate days, and Jean, who died in 1980 and was the catalyst for my entry into the field of biomedical ethics, was my mother. These cases, and many others like them that I have encountered in my hospice and hospital work, have taught me that the practice of medicine and health care cannot be limited to the treatment of disease and illness. It needs to include a component that directly addresses the holistic human and emotional requirements of both the patient and the patient's family, and it must consciously address ethical and moral principles that affect health care actions and options.

It is my belief that this need can be addressed through biomedical ethics education. Such education can directly provide workers in the medical community with information not only about biomedical ethics in general but also about how to apply that knowledge in actual situations.

This book has been developed as a resource to be used in the planning and application of biomedical ethics education. The major objectives of the book are to provide an overview of a comprehensive biomedical ethics education program, basic information concerning the general field of biomedical ethics, and a wide variety of resources that can be used in biomedical ethics education programs and events. The book is intended as a planning instrument for the individual who is new to biomedical ethics education and as a reference tool for the experienced educator who is looking for ways to enhance an existing program.

Although this book is not intended to address all of the subject matter pertaining to biomedical ethics or to include all possible activities that could be included in a biomedical ethics education program, it does cover several key elements that would be appropriate to include in such a program. These elements are:

- Guidance on the development of a scope and sequence for a biomedical ethics education program, including a rationale for the inclusion of *all* staff members in the plan
- An overview of biomedical ethics issues and topics
- A strategy for the development of a process for ethical thinking and review
- Information on the steps needed to develop and conduct a grand rounds program in biomedical ethics
- A selection of educational tools, such as role plays, structured learning activities, and case studies, that can be used to reinforce conceptual knowledge and provide experience in the practical application of skills

It is my hope that this book will be a useful instrument for educators, members of biomedical ethics committees, and administrators as they develop and conduct educational programs that will enable health care workers to understand and address ethical issues.

Acknowledgments

This book would not have been possible without the assistance and support of many individuals. I wish to thank:

- Fr. Fred Tillitson, director of ethics for the Franciscan Health System, for the wealth of information and ethical expertise that he has provided
- Richard Hill, my editor at American Hospital Publishing, Inc., for his belief in the value of this endeavor and for his excellent advice and guidance
- Dr. Bruce Uhrich, my friend and colleague, for his moral support, and for his skillful review and advice on the content of the book
- Dr. Edwin R. Knopf for being my mentor and guide throughout the years of my professional life

And special, sincere, thanks goes to my family, for their constant patience, encouragement, and understanding.

Chapter One

Introduction to Biomedical Ethics Education

The purpose of biomedical ethics education is to facilitate a relationship between ethical theory and the practical application of that theory in real-life situations. Ultimately, the goal of biomedical ethics education is to improve the knowledge base of the participants to ensure that the highest standards of practice will be used in the provision of physical and emotional care to terminally and critically ill patients. (See figure 1-1.)

The Value and Purpose of Biomedical Ethics Education

In a practical sense, biomedical ethics education provides valuable opportunities for participants to:

- Learn about specific information concerning the field of biomedical ethics and about policies, cases, situations, and medical advances that have an ethical component
- Explore various philosophical and theoretical points of view
- Learn the vocabulary and terminology used in ethical discussions
- Clarify personal values
- Listen to the opinions and beliefs of others
- Develop and enhance communication skills
- Practice the art of logical reasoning
- Identify resources available for additional learning
- Develop respect for, and an understanding of, the multidimensional, interdisciplinary roles that combine to provide compassionate, high-quality holistic patient care

A good educational setting also provides a safe environment where participants can discuss and question a biomedical ethics dilemma and, in some cases, challenge the rationale for specific courses of action.

Figure 1-1. The Purpose of Biomedical Ethics Education

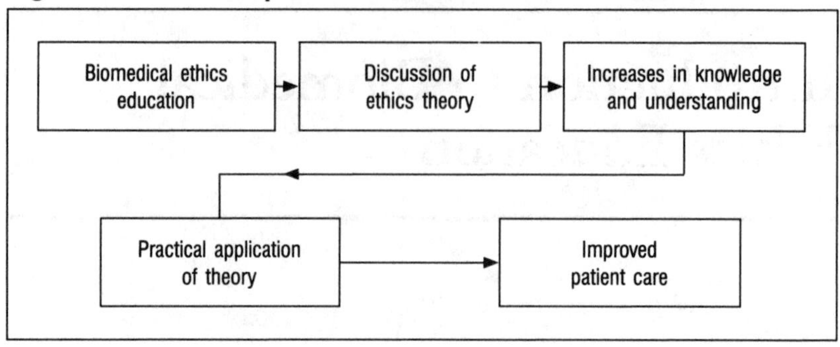

Formalized biomedical ethics education can, over time, encourage and promote real and observable changes in a health care setting, including the following:

- *Informal discussions:* Individuals who have participated in biomedical ethics education activities are more likely than others to have the knowledge, confidence, and desire to initiate and conduct informal discussions about ethical issues and problematic cases. These informal discussions have the potential to improve communication between the patient, the family, and the physicians and also to involve in ethical issues a wider variety of providers from other disciplines within the health care setting.
- *Case consultations:* Biomedical ethics education promotes a level of awareness that fosters referrals to the biomedical ethics committee (or other appropriate group) for prospective case consultation. Once individuals are comfortable with a structured case review process (see chapter 4) and the value of that process is recognized, the advantages of referring cases to a committee for guidance become apparent.
- *Awareness of options:* Informed decision making concerning medical care requires that all available options be known and understood. Biomedical ethics education serves to keep participants as up-to-date as possible on the current thinking, risks, and benefits about available treatments and options. Once participants are aware of these options, they will be better prepared to provide this information to patients and their family members and can consequently assist in the application of this knowledge in practical situations.
- *Demystification:* For many years, ethics has been perceived as being in the realm of philosophers and theologians. The need to assimilate ethical understanding and thinking into the everyday practice of medicine, by all health care workers, was largely unrecognized. Biomedical ethics education can reduce outdated perceptions and thus bring a comfort level about ethics to a broader base of individuals.
- *Outreach:* Besides promoting an understanding of the various components of biomedical ethics among all health care workers, biomedical ethics education

can extend far beyond the hospital walls to provide both opportunity and information to the lay community. By providing education on health care topics, information about treatment risks and benefits, and advice about patients' advance directives, the health care facility's staff can help the community become better equipped to ask appropriate questions, gather needed information, and ultimately make informed health care decisions.

What Biomedical Ethics Education Is, and What It Is Not

Ethics is not a new subject. Throughout medical history there have been codes of practice, recognized standards of care, and a progression of public policy, human involvement, and ideas that have had ethical components. Ethics has always provided a framework for health care treatments and decisions.

In the past two decades, major changes in medicine have resulted in vast growth in the field of biomedical ethics. This growth has occurred in the frequency and type of issues that have an ethical implication and in the formalization of educational efforts designed to provide health care professionals with information and tools to understand and deal with ethical issues. There also has been a growing trend toward expanded awareness of ethics and an apparent thirst for knowledge about the topic of ethics among health care workers and private citizens.

As this awareness has expanded, so too have the need and desire for education that will enable interested individuals to approach ethical issues with a uniform knowledge base and a consistent process for reflection, discussion, and interpretation. Biomedical ethics education has developed as a formal and informal vehicle through which an individual, team, or committee can examine, assess, review, and discuss the total field of biomedical ethics and the moral principles and values that influence the practice of health care.

Historically, the vast amount of ethics education relating to medicine has taken place in formal settings such as colleges and universities or in medical and nursing schools.[1] Today, biomedical ethics education also takes place in hospitals, nursing homes, hospices, community centers, and sometimes in the public media. It is now recognized that for biomedical ethics education to be effective and comprehensive, it must not only be provided to trained medical practitioners but must also expand the circle of participants to include members of institutional biomedical ethics committees, staff members from ancillary departments within the institution, public-policy makers, and concerned members of the general public.[2]

In hospital settings, the effect of biomedical ethics education can be enhanced by making educational experiences both interdisciplinary and interdepartmental. The goal of this effort should be to make ethical thinking a conscious component of every aspect of the care provided. This goal can be reached only if all members of the hospital staff are given the opportunity to develop a familiarity and a comfort level with ethics in general and with biomedical ethics in particular.

On the other hand, biomedical ethics education is *not* a specific program. It does not consist only of identified, clearly defined blocks of information or activities that are standardized and easily replicated. Nevertheless, there are some consistent components to biomedical ethics education. These components should ideally constitute the building blocks of any educational effort. The building blocks (figure 1-2) should be integrated into a process that is adaptable to changes in medical technology, the passage of ethics-related legislation, the impact of court decisions, and the ebb and flow of the human and cultural context of the issues at hand.

Biomedical ethics education is not a forum in which to discuss health care *business* ethics. Although there are basic ethical principles and values that have an impact on business decisions, contracts, conflicts of interest, and so on, these are not a component of biomedical ethics and are best addressed in another setting.

Most important, biomedical ethics education should not be used as a way to promote change to a certain way of thinking or to a certain belief system. It should also not be used to encourage the adoption of a particular point of view. Furthermore, it is not the role of biomedical ethics educators to influence the course of any particular health care decision.

Figure 1-2. Building Blocks of Biomedical Ethics Education

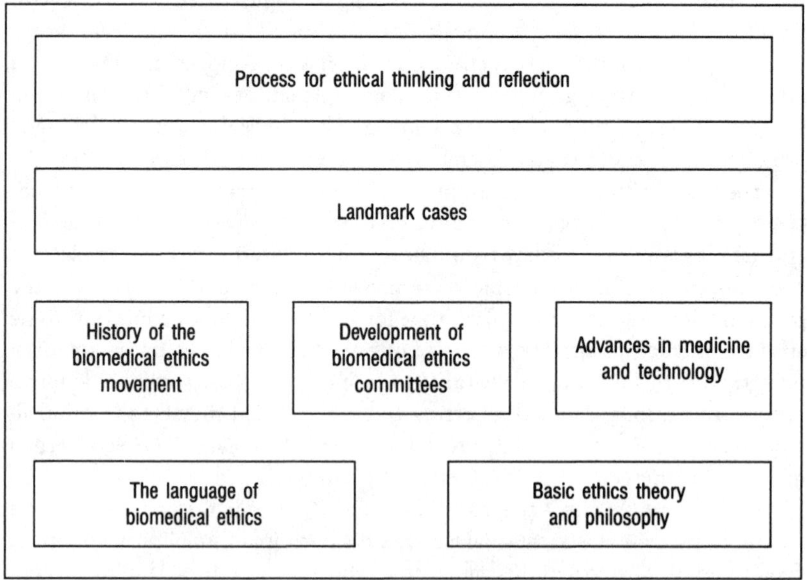

Developing a Mind-Set

The most important factor that distinguishes biomedical ethics from any other aspect of medicine or health care is that ethics and ethical issues permeate every aspect of everything done with and for a patient. Whether or not we realize it, no option is offered, no decision is made, and no treatment or procedure is performed without addressing the question, Is this the right thing to do? In many cases, the answer is an unqualified yes. When everyone agrees, there naturally is no conflict. In some instances, however, the answer is not so obvious, and the need to explore the situation from an ethical perspective arises.

Clearly, this is not always an easy thing to do. The answer to what is the "right" thing to do may differ greatly, depending on who is asked. Because individuals who work in health care settings come from different philosophical, theological, and sociocultural backgrounds, this creates an institutional matrix of ethical thinking, which is complex indeed.

It is therefore important for any biomedical ethics education process to work toward the establishment of a mind-set within the institution. This mind-set not only should promote an obligation to openly identify the ethical components of patient interactions, but also should recognize that differences of opinion among the participants in any discussion are appropriate and accepted. To promote a positive institutional mind-set for the acceptance and integration of biomedical ethics education, it is useful for the educator to be aware of certain basic assumptions—about the adult learner and about the topic of ethics—that will have an impact on this educational process.

Assumptions about the Adult Learner

Biomedical ethics educators should make certain assumptions about adult learners. These assumptions include the following:

- Adults learn best when the educational experience in which they are participating is nonauthoritarian, informal, and interactive.
- Each individual adult learner comes to an experience with a different background, different expectations of what the program can provide, and varied learning needs and capacities.
- Although individuals continue to learn throughout their lives, the adult learner will approach an experience more positively if direct benefits of the expected learning are readily apparent and if the experience is likely to result in personal benefit.
- Adults tend to approach new learning experiences with some anxiety. They may be reluctant to openly explore new topics. This is especially true when the topic is in any way threatening or controversial.

- Adults learn best when they participate in the learning process. Active learning enables a participant to assimilate a larger amount of information than passive learning does.
- Nonjudgmental, positive feedback to participants will reinforce learning that has taken place and will heighten the perception of a worthwhile experience, thus setting the stage for additional learning in any future programs.

Assumptions about the Topic of Ethics

Biomedical ethics educators should also be aware of assumptions about the topic of ethics in general. Following are some of these assumptions:

- Ethics is abstract, biased, subjective, and emotional. Individuals generally perceive themselves to be ethical.
- Ethical beliefs are based on values that are highly personal, powerful, and deeply ingrained. Expressed differences in personal values are likely to cause some level of conflict.
- Biomedical ethics is a subject rich in cultural, political, social, and religious diversity. Total agreement by every participant in a discussion is virtually impossible.
- Consensus has not been reached on the exact meaning of many of the terms used in the discussion of biomedical ethics. Terms such as *quality of life*, *informed consent*, or *ordinary/extraordinary care* are not quantifiable and, as such, leave room for various interpretations.
- Information and opinions about topics in the field of biomedical ethics are constantly changing and expanding. Any discussion related to any aspect of biomedical ethics is likely to generate more questions than answers.

The Language of Biomedical Ethics

All fields of study have a specialized and unique vocabulary. Although biomedical ethics is part of the larger specialty of medicine and although some medical practitioners may be familiar with the language of ethics, many of the words used in the discussion of biomedical ethics topics are *not* typical of general medical terminology. Therefore, it is important for any biomedical ethics education effort to include information about the meanings of words and phrases as they are used in an ethical context.

It is especially important to provide information about ethics terminology when educational efforts expand to include an interdisciplinary audience. Individuals who are not physicians or nurses are less likely to have a background in ethics language than medical professionals are and therefore would need this information as a framework for learning.

The glossary at the end of this book includes many of the words and phrases that are likely to be encountered in the study of biomedical ethics. This list does not, however, include all of the possible terms that may enter into a biomedical ethics discussion. Additional information or clarification may be helpful to individuals learning about this subject.

As the general knowledge about biomedical ethics grows and changes from year to year, so too will the words and phrases used to describe the discipline. Institutions that provide ethics education have an obligation to keep current with these changes and to provide staff with up-to-date information.

Summary

The future issues surrounding biomedical ethics are unclear and will depend largely on changes in the medical field, such as advances in technology, knowledge of diseases and cures, and changes in the national health care delivery system. It is clear, however, that biomedical ethics will continue to have an important role in the health care setting. The role of biomedical ethics education will continue to be a vital one, providing the link between knowledge and facts as well as practical application in the effort to make appropriate and informed health care decisions. This role is likely to expand as patients, family caregivers, and service providers become more aware of their options, of their individual human values, and of the collective social conscience, all of which influence the provision of health care.

References

1. Coutts, M. C. Teaching ethics in the health care setting. Part 1: survey of the literature. *Kennedy Institute of Ethics Journal* 16(2):171–85, June 1991.
2. Thornton, B. C., Callahan, D., and Nelson, J. Bioethics education: expanding the circle of participants. *Hastings Center Report* 23(1):25–29, Jan.–Feb. 1993.

Suggested Readings

Bernat, J. The boundaries of the persistent vegetative state. *Journal of Clinical Ethics* 3(3):167–80, Fall 1992.

Emanuel, E. J., and Emanuel, L. C. Proxy decision making for incompetent patients. *JAMA* 267(15):2067–71, Apr. 15, 1992.

deBlois, J. Ethical issues in healthcare: informed consent and the purpose of medicine. *Center for Healthcare Ethics* 12(6):1–2, Feb. 1991.

Sanders, L. M., and Raffin, T. A. The ethics of withholding and withdrawing critical care. *Cambridge Quarterly of Healthcare Ethics* 2:175–84, 1993.

Veatch, R. Brain death and slippery slopes. *Journal of Clinical Ethics* 3(3):181–87, Fall 1992.

Wax, J. Defining ethical and avoiding dilemmas. *Hospital Ethics* 7(6):12–14, Nov.–Dec. 1991.

Chapter Two

The Scope and Sequence of Biomedical Ethics Education

In a health care setting, there are four target groups for biomedical ethics education:

- The biomedical ethics committee
- The professional and clinical staff
- The nonprofessional and nonclinical staff
- The community

Although each group is distinct and approaches biomedical ethics education from its own perspective and with specific learning needs, a basic knowledge of biomedical ethics and an understanding of ethical issues are equally important for all groups.

Developing an Interdisciplinary Strategy

Because of the complexity of biomedical ethics and the vast amount of subject matter in the field, an institution conducting biomedical ethics education would be wise to work from a cautious and systematic implementation plan. The plan should continuously expand to include new groups of participants and new educational experiences. As groups are added to the matrix, the preceding groups should continue their own educational efforts and become incorporated into the new group. Any attempt to educate all groups simultaneously is likely to cause more confusion than understanding.

This is not to say that biomedical ethics education has a beginning and an end—that one group finishes and another group starts. On the contrary, biomedical ethics education never ends. The learning is ongoing and constantly changing, with different groups at different points along a continuum of learning at any moment in time. By starting formalized educational efforts with one group and then expanding the effort to include other groups at a later time, an institution encourages the development of a strong ethics foundation, which will help foster the integration of ethics awareness and thinking for both interdisciplinary and interdepartmental audiences.

Once a perceived comfort level has been reached within an institution, biomedical ethics education efforts can then be expanded beyond the staff to include professional and lay members of the general community. Groups such as students, the clergy, volunteers, and senior citizens would benefit from programs designed to increase their understanding of biomedical ethics. Such outreach efforts not only benefit community audiences but also enhance institutional understanding by bringing additional opportunities for reflection and alternative perspectives into the educational matrix. Figure 2-1 illustrates the incorporation phases of groups from the biomedical ethics committee out to the community-at-large.

Comprehensive biomedical ethics education is a lengthy process, and this must be considered in the strategic planning of any programs. Figure 2-2 presents a suggested time frame for ethics education.

Defining the Biomedical Ethics Committee

The logical place to begin any educational effort on the topic of biomedical ethics is with the biomedical ethics committee. Members of this committee have made a commitment to become involved in institutionwide ethical issues and

Figure 2-1. Phases of Biomedical Ethics Education

Phase IV

Phase III

Phase II

Phase I

The biomedical ethics committee

The professional staff

The nonprofessional staff

The community

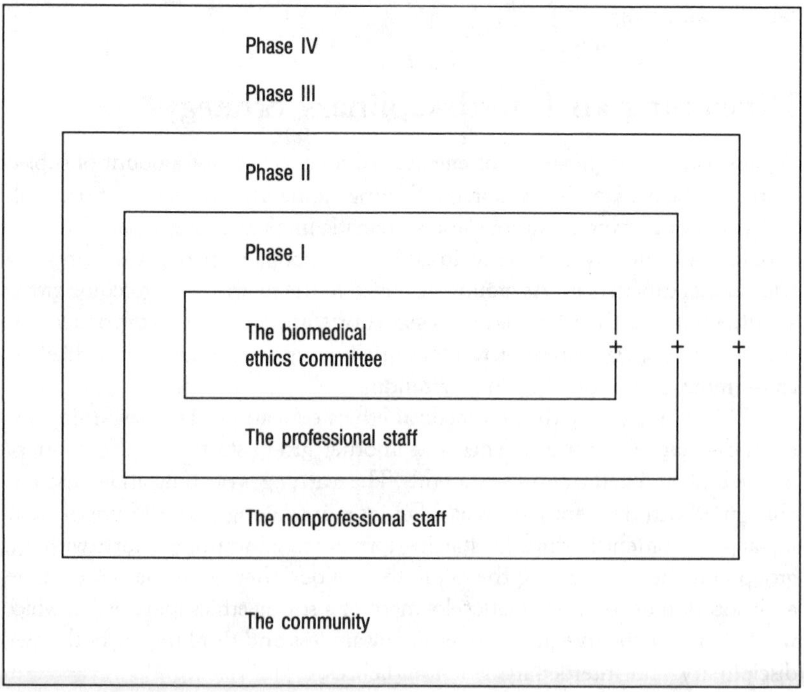

Figure 2-2. Suggested Time Frame for Ethics Education

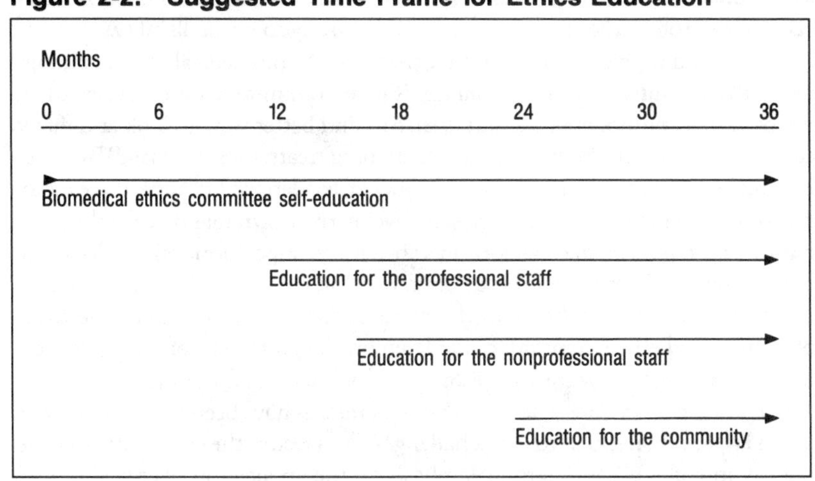

must have a working knowledge of ethics in general and the impact that ethical issues can have on patient care.

The biomedical ethics committee is the core group for any biomedical ethics effort within a health care facility, and its members play a key role in discussions of ethical dimensions in patient care. The following subsections discuss the evolution of biomedical ethics committees, committee members and their roles, and the education of the committee.

The Evolution of Biomedical Ethics Committees

The development of biomedical ethics committees began in the 1960s, when some states required that hospitals address specific medical issues and problems through a committee format. For example, committees were established to decide which patient/candidate would receive limited dialysis resources or whether an abortion could be performed legally. Later, infant care committees were established in neonatal intensive care units in response to the "Baby Doe" regulations developed under the Reagan administration.[1]

Two other types of committees were precursors to the modern biomedical ethics committee. *The institutional review board (IRB),* also known as the *human studies committee* or the *human subjects committee,* is a long-standing type of committee that oversees research on human subjects. It was established and is governed by federal law. Any proposed research involving human subjects must be reviewed by an IRB before the start of the study and before any potential subjects are recruited. The IRB also functions as a safeguard to ensure that the interests of the patients/research subjects are protected (for example, through the use of informed consent, through the provision of adequate information, and by ensuring that no "rewards" are being offered for the assumption of risks).

The primary function of an IRB is not necessarily to make research more ethical but to protect the institution from any wrongdoing or liability.

A second type of committee that predates the biomedical ethics committee is the *institutional ethics committee*. These committees were developed in response to institutional needs and desires to find better ways to look at difficult cases, particularly those involving life-sustaining treatments. Unlike IRBs, these committees are not governed by specific laws or regulations but instead are established by individual institutions, which develop their own mandate for the committee and establish the mission, membership composition, and tasks to be accomplished. What makes these committees different from biomedical ethics committees is their emphasis on the word *institutional*. Historically, the focus of institutional ethics committees has been on the protection of the institution from future litigation by the establishment of policies and forums for case review.

The main tasks of institutional ethics committees have been to review changes in the law and to respond to legal challenges. As a result, these committees have not traditionally placed a strong emphasis on the application of ethical theory or on the development of ethics education. Biomedical ethics committees, on the other hand, tend to take a broader approach to the subject of ethics and emphasize the needs of the patient and the staff as well as those of the institution.

In some institutions that have had an institutional ethics committee for a long time, the committee has evolved and now has a mission similar to that of a biomedical ethics committee; however, the name "institutional ethics committee" has remained the same. In some hospitals the committee name has simply been shortened to "ethics committee." It is important, therefore, to look at not only the name of a committee but also the identity that the committee has established and the tasks and activities that members of the committee perform.

Part of the identity that the committee establishes will be a function of the body that mandates the committee's existence. (See figure 2-3.) The biomedical ethics committee can be a committee appointed by the institution's governing board or administration, or it can be a medical staff committee. The committee's function and role in the institution will be determined by how the committee has been established and by its place in the overall organizational structure.

The membership composition of the biomedical ethics committee will vary greatly, depending on the needs of the institution. In some cases, the committee may be made up largely of physicians. This is particularly true when the committee is part of the medical staff structure. In other cases, there may be minimal physician representation.

Also, in the early stages of committee development, the membership may be composed of individuals who are handpicked to frame the activities of the committee. As the value to and reputation of the committee grows within the institution, other individuals may become interested in the work of the committee and wish to volunteer to serve on it. As such, there may be a need to review and change the membership composition on a regular basis.

Figure 2-3. Examples of Models for Organizational Placement of a Biomedical Ethics Committee

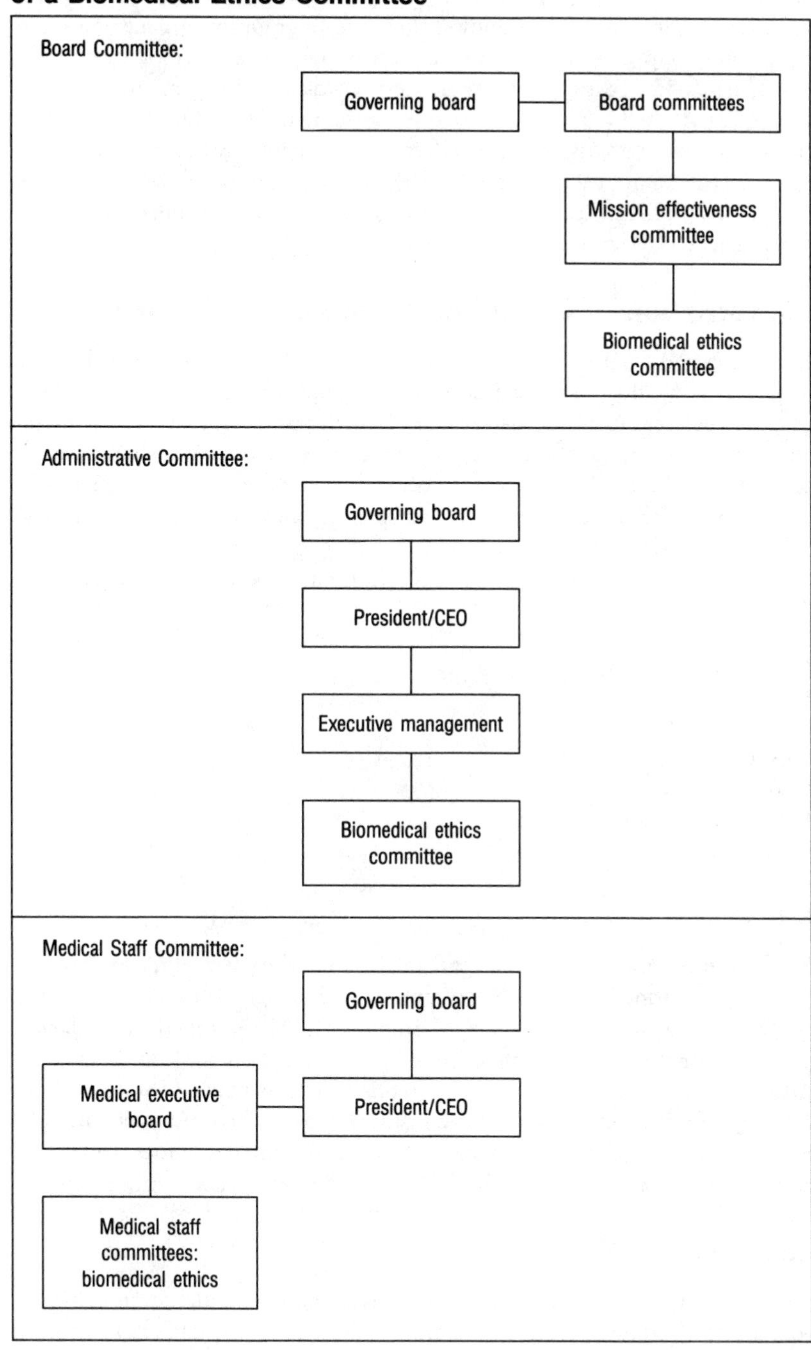

In some institutions, all members of the biomedical ethics committee, including the chairperson, are appointed for a specific time period. In other institutions, there may be a standing chair with a group of core members and a separate group of members who rotate through on a specified schedule.

The individual designated to chair the biomedical ethics committee will vary, depending on the function of the body that has mandated that the committee exists. If the committee is a medical staff committee, it is likely that a physician will chair it. If the committee was established by the governing body or administration, the chair may be a physician, but it is just as likely that someone from another discipline, such as social services, pastoral care, or nursing, will assume the responsibility.

A Description of Committee Members and Their Roles

The number of committee members and their job titles are determined by the needs of the facility. Each institution has an obligation to recruit individuals who are interested in ethics, are respected in their positions, and can help establish or enhance the credibility of the committee. All participants should clearly define and understand the roles of the committee members. All members should be able to bring both knowledge of their specialty and a unique personal viewpoint to the committee discussions.

Some typical committee members and their respective roles (detailed in the following subsections) are:

- Administrator
- Community member
- Nurse
- Educator
- Ethicist
- Pastoral care staff member
- Physician
- Lawyer
- Social worker

It is important to note that part of the role of each committee member is to share information from the committee with others. It may take time for new committee members to feel comfortable with biomedical ethics, and even more time for them to feel confident enough to share this knowledge in another setting, but a committee that never extends its efforts beyond the committee meeting is of little or no value to the institution as a whole. As such, an obligation to assist with both formal and informal educational activities is an essential component of the role of each of the biomedical ethics committee members.

Administrator

A representative of the institution's administration is essential to provide support to the committee.[2] The biomedical ethics committee must have at least one administrator as well as a powerful representative of the medical services staff to ensure overall credibility and maintain authority to implement plans and programs. When a committee lacks this support and is only made up of interested, well-intended individuals, the mechanisms for action may be compromised.

Community Member

A layperson from the community who sits on a biomedical ethics committee brings to the committee the point of view of a health care consumer. This individual approaches discussions from a nonclinical and nontrained point of view and is likely to raise questions that a "medically aware" group might not consider. Lay individuals on a biomedical ethics committee should be representative of the community in which the facility is located. This could be somewhat problematic in that most, if not all, communities are made up of many different demographic characteristics (race and ethnicity, age, income level, and so on). Selection of community members who represent all of these demographic characteristics would be neither possible nor wise. Care must be taken to select a community member who is able to share his or her perspective as well as exhibit an awareness of the multidimensional aspects of the community as a whole.

Nurse

The nursing staff should be well represented on a biomedical ethics committee. As direct caregivers, nurses often have greater contact with the patient, the family, and significant others than any other group within the health care setting. As such, they are aware of conflicts surrounding specific treatment decisions and of ethical problems that arise concerning treatment and patient care. Although in the day-to-day working environment, nurses are in a position to observe, question, and assist, they frequently are not in a position to challenge the authority of others. Representatives of nursing administration, critical care, cardiac care, neonatal intensive care, and the medical and surgical units can bring a unique perspective to the committee.

Educator

A representative of the institution's education department should serve on the committee. This representative helps guide committee members in the development and continuation of their own education. Additionally, this individual assists in the development and execution of a plan of action to carry the committee's message to a broader audience. The educator's responsibilities can include providing resources and tools for the committee to use, developing and reviewing specific educational materials, and conducting educational activities and programs (both internal and external to the committee) that focus on ethics and ethical issues. In addition, the educator can assist in planning outreach activities for community audiences.

Ethicist

An ethicist who serves on a biomedical ethics committee acts primarily as a resource for the committee members by offering guidance in the processes of ethical thinking and reflection. In some institutions, such as teaching hospitals, the ethicist may be part of the staff. In other institutions, the ethicist is likely to be from the outside—from a college or university, for example. The role of the ethicist is neither to draw conclusions nor to provide moral judgments. Instead, the ethicist should guide the committee in the analysis of ethical situations and help members look at the medical and clinical components of a case from the perspective of ethics and ethical philosophy.

Pastoral Care Staff Member

Hospital pastoral care staff members and chaplains bring to the committee an awareness and consciousness of religious issues that arise concerning ethical issues and choices. These issues arise among committee members and in real-life cases. The different religious backgrounds of the committee members undoubtedly affect how they view particular issues. It is the role of the pastoral care member to assist other committee members in identifying religious issues that may be causing conflict. In addition, the pastoral care member should be available as a resource for guidance in obtaining information on different faiths. This individual can also be a vehicle for outreach to various clergy members within the community.

Physician

An effective biomedical ethics committee needs to have several physician members. In many institutions, the number of physicians is approximately one-third to one-half of the total membership. Representation of physicians from a number of different specialties is ideal; family practice, cardiology, oncology, neonatology, and internal medicine are frequently represented. Physicians, of course, approach ethical discussions from a clinical and medical point of view. As the climate of medical practice evolves and as changes in health care delivery occur, physician input into the ethical dimension of practice will continue to be vital. In addition, significant physician involvement with the committee brings additional credibility to the work of the committee and can be an important link between the committee and other physicians on staff. Physicians can act as a resource for clinical and patient-related information on an established ethical review process (see chapter 4) and can also encourage other physicians to refer difficult situations to the ethics committee for prospective case consultation.

Lawyer

A lawyer on the committee may be the hospital's legal counsel or the risk manager (if that individual is also a lawyer). The role of the lawyer on a biomedical ethics committee is to advise the committee on what is *safe* and legally sound for the institution, the patients, and members of the committee. The lawyer keeps committee members aware of changes in laws and regulations, pending court cases, and precedents concerning specific cases and issues and informs them of legal issues that might affect the deliberations, discussions, and decisions of the committee. In addition, the lawyer acts as a resource in policy development and revision, suggesting new policies that would assist the institution in the practical application of ethical theory. Some health care institutions also have a lawyer on the committee who is not an employee of the institution. Such an appointment is designed to prevent conflicts of interest, which may arise if there is a disagreement between the institution and a patient or a patient's decision maker.

Social Worker

The social worker on the committee brings to the discussions a perspective that examines the patient and the ethical situation from a holistic psychosocial viewpoint. The social worker can address short- and long-range implications as well as the complex family dimensions of an issue. This individual is adept at integrating the medical aspects of a situation with cultural, societal, and family components.

The Education of the Committee

A biomedical ethics committee bears little resemblance to most other committees in an institutional setting. The main goals of this committee are to provide opportunities for combining theory with process and to foster an understanding of the relationship between actions and moral principles. Unlike other committees, the biomedical ethics committee does not strive to make operational a business component of health care. Therefore, by its very nature, this committee regularly faces numerous problems, complex issues, and unique opportunities. The actions and deliberations of the committee are more open-ended than those of other committees and consequently more problematic to define. Given the constantly evolving knowledge base of biomedical ethics and the state of flux that defines the very existence of a biomedical ethics committee, it is easy to see why the task of educating committee members is, at best, time-consuming, difficult, and challenging.

Education for members of a biomedical ethics committee includes two major phases:

- The initial (or orientation) phase
- The ongoing (or enrichment) phase

The methods employed in each phase are a function of the design of the committee, the stage that the committee is in with regard to its historical development, and the committee membership composition and tenure schedule.

The Initial (Orientation) Phase

Every new committee must have a starting point. This is called the *initial* (or *orientation*) *phase.* The impetus for the development of a biomedical ethics committee can come from several sources. They include an administrative request, physician need, regulatory requirements, staff interest in biomedical ethics, and reformulation of an existing committee to take on a more in-depth ethics focus.

Once it has been established that there will be a biomedical ethics committee, it is necessary to identify well-respected individuals who are interested in the topic of ethics, willing to serve on the committee, and able to assume the responsibility for establishing a structure for the new committee. As this initial committee develops, its members will need to learn about biomedical ethics in general. They will also need to learn specifically about their roles and functions related to the institution in order to develop the groundwork for the biomedical ethics committee and set the educational foundation for future committee members.

When it is established, a biomedical ethics committee usually has three main functions: policy development and review, outreach education, and case review and consultation. A new committee must plan how it will accomplish each of these functions. A committee's strategic plan must identify the scope of each area and the projected implementation schedule of activities that will support the functions. Before undertaking these tasks, the committee must engage in an extensive period of self-education. This is necessary in order for members to develop a common base from which to work as they subsequently deliberate issues and then begin to broaden their efforts and activities throughout the institution.

Resources such as the *Handbook for Hospital Ethics Committees*[3] and *Biomedical Ethics*[4] are practical guides for the planning and development of a new committee and can provide valuable, basic information about the field of biomedical ethics. Use of these books and other resources can help form a consistent knowledge base and provide a framework for the development of cohesiveness among the new committee members.

The committee members must also decide which specific areas of ethics and biomedical ethics are important to their mission *and* the needs of the institution. They must identify sources that can provide them with the information that they think is needed about those areas. This fact-finding task can be intimidating and confusing, given the huge amount of material available. Careful and selective literature searches and a deliberate planning, review, and recommendation process will greatly assist in meeting this goal. In some cases, an informational discussion about specific topics will be held during the meetings of the committee. In other cases (particularly when a committee member has an identified need or a personal interest in a topic), continuing education will be carried out apart from the committee setting.

The initial self-education of a new biomedical ethics committee takes a great deal of time, perhaps a year or more. Any attempt to move beyond the self-education stage into policy development, outreach education, or case consultation before the committee feels that it is adequately educated in the basics of ethical theory, ethics terminology, and bioethical history will result in weaknesses in those areas, which may ultimately compromise the group's effectiveness.

It is unlikely that the individuals who are initially appointed to the biomedical ethics committee will remain on the committee permanently. Indeed, one of the first tasks that a new committee must accomplish is to decide how the committee tenure and membership rotation will be structured.

Some possible models of biomedical ethics committees include the following:

- A committee that has an identified core group of members (frequently five or six members of the original committee) who remain on the committee at all times. Other members are appointed for two-year or three-year terms, staggered so that a new group of members replaces a portion of the rotating membership every year.
- A committee wherein all members are appointed for specific periods and are replaced when their term expires.
- A committee wherein all members are appointed for undefined terms and are replaced only if they resign from the committee.

Each committee model has its own unique advantages and disadvantages, and no particular model is necessarily the best. However, no matter which model is adopted, the task of providing the educational framework for any new member of the committee is difficult. As previously stated, there needs to be considerable time and effort spent in educating biomedical ethics committee members. The challenge becomes how to add new members to the committee and bring them up-to-date without spending all of the committee's meeting time on educational efforts and without repeating information and previous discussions.

One possible solution to this problem is to have the committee develop its own internal resource for committee orientation. A loose-leaf notebook could be amended and updated periodically and given to each new committee member. Ideally, new members would enter as a group, and a full-day seminar would be conducted. During the seminar, discussions based on the content of the orientation book would be led by the committee chair or the educator on the committee. Alternatively, an orientation book could be given to each new member at the time he or she joins. (In such cases, follow-up and review by the chair or the educator is recommended.)

Topics appropriate for an orientation book include:

- Mission and goals of the committee
- Names and job titles of the existing members
- Roles and responsibilities of the members
- General information on group process:
  - Leadership theory
  - Rules of the committee
  - Participation guidelines
  - Conflict resolution
  - Prioritization of tasks
- Definitions of the basic terms encountered in the study of ethics
- Basic theoretical foundations:
  - Moral principles
  - Ethical principles
- Summary of the history of the bioethics movement
- Outline of a process used for ethical thinking and reflection
- History of the committee:
  - List of major tasks and accomplishments
  - Conflicts that have been addressed
  - Summary of educational programs previously conducted (including copies of handouts and educational materials)
- Copies of existing policies related to ethical issues
- List of policies currently in development
- List of books, journal articles, and other resources recommended for additional learning and in-depth study of ethical issues

Although biomedical ethics committees have the potential to make significant contributions, many have fallen into dangerous territory by not clearly establishing a committee identity, a method of action, or a place for the committee within the institution. As a result, the committee may lack credibility, and committee members—who may have been inspired and energized in the beginning—may lose interest or believe that their time is not being well spent. Therefore, it is essential for members of a new committee to be as specific as possible concerning the reasons that the committee exists, the actions the committee plans to take, and the process by which those actions are to be undertaken.

The Ongoing (Enrichment) Phase

In addition to providing orientation for each new member of a biomedical ethics committee, it is necessary to provide continuing education so that committee members can remain up-to-date on the factors that affect the field. This is the *ongoing* (or *enrichment*) *phase*.

Several methods can be employed to facilitate ongoing education. The most obvious method is to include an educational component on the agenda for each committee meeting. Topics for this agenda item might include:

- Ethical issues or cases in the news
- New laws and regulations that will influence ethical decision making
- Pending court decisions concerning treatment issues
- Health care and medical advances that may pose an ethical dilemma
- Allocation of resources: debates and decisions

A second method of providing continuing education for members of the biomedical ethics committee is to arrange for them to attend conferences, seminars, or courses specializing in an ethics or biomedical ethics topic. Many such opportunities are offered at hospitals and medical centers as well as through institutions of higher learning. These opportunities can be valuable in that they not only provide the chance for attendees to learn new information but also offer the occasion for committee members to network with other people who are interested or experienced in the subject. They can be helpful in validating the accomplishments of the committee, in gathering new ideas and suggestions, and in identifying some of the common difficulties that committees have.

A third method for continuing the education of members of a biomedical ethics committee is through the provision of books, articles, videos, and other resources. Because a vast quantity of ethics information is available, it is critical for the committee to be selective in choosing materials to distribute, so as not to overwhelm its members. In addition, a significant amount of such material focuses on a particular viewpoint and attempts to convince the reader or viewer to adopt a certain position or opinion. It is essential for the committee to be aware of these possible biases and to select materials that will provide members with information about all sides of an issue.

Once the committee feels that it has a solid educational base from which to work, then—and only then—should it begin to focus on the specific tasks for which it was created. Often, the committee begins its work with the development or revision of policies that have an ethical component or implication. Although by no means inclusive of every possible policy that an ethics committee might consider or develop, the following are some of the most likely policies to be brought to the table:

- Adoption
- Advance directives
- Anatomical gift
- Confidentiality
- Consent for human immunodeficiency virus (HIV) antibody testing
- Corneas, procurement of, and care of donors
- Dignity of the deceased

- Informed consent for diagnostic workup or medical treatment
- Informed consent for surgery
- Life-support choices for the dying patient
- "No code" or do-not-resuscitate (DNR) orders for inpatients
- Patient rights and responsibilities
- Postmortem examination and authorization
- Process for ethical consultation and guidance
- Rape
- Termination of pregnancy
- Use of restraints

As policies are finalized and approved, the committee should make certain that the policy information is adequately disseminated to the staff. This, in all likelihood, will be the first of the formal educational efforts for the committee.

Broadening the Educational Experience

Assuming that ethics education is one of the identified functions of the biomedical ethics committee, the next step, after members have engaged in adequate self-education, is for members to expand their efforts and share their knowledge with other staff members.

Some questions to address in relation to this task are as follows:

- What is the best way to reach these audiences?
- What information is necessary for the staff members to have?
- What is the appropriate scope and sequence?
- How can the vast amount of knowledge in the field of ethics be made meaningful to a diverse audience?

Although the details of these questions are best answered within the institution where the ethics education will take place, some generic, global answers apply to most settings.

Many health care institutions already have a mechanism in place for the continuing education of the professional staff. Continuing medical education (CME) programs are offered in cooperation with medical schools and universities, and educational in-service programs are offered to staff by education and training departments and through nursing education. When possible, ethics education can be included in these schedules.

To enhance the exchange of information, guest speakers can be invited from the community or videos can be used. Small discussion groups that address a specific topic or journal clubs can also be used. Some institutions participate in formal ethics education programs,[5] such as "Decisions near the End of Life," which provide structured opportunities to address specific areas of learning.

Another method of providing ethics education is through ethics grand rounds programs. (See chapter 5.) These programs enable participants to observe and participate in the process of ethics deliberation and provide staff with a broad mix of ethics theory with a framework for practical application.

The following sections discuss ethics education for the professional staff and the nonprofessional staff, integration of biomedical ethics education into other institutional activities, and the extension of biomedical ethics education to the community.

Ethics Education for the Professional Staff

For the purposes of this book, the professional staff is identified as a group of individuals who have had formal training in a medical, clinical, or other organized health care discipline. It is assumed that, in the course of their training, these individuals would have had some exposure to medical ethics or at least to health care decision making.

Professional staff members include:

- Health care administrators
- Cardiopulmonary specialists
- Health educators
- Nurses
- Pastoral care staff
- Physicians
- Rehabilitation services staff
- Social workers

Professional staff members need to know ethics information that they can use to help their patients and themselves identify and deal with ethical problems and conflicts. They need to know policies, laws, and regulations as well as those more subtle human, emotional, and moral or value-laden factors on which health care decisions and desires are based.

Health care professionals also need to know what to do, and how to do it, should they become involved in a situation about which they need specific guidance. Information on the role of the ethics committee, how to access the committee, and the process that the committee uses to provide case review should be presented and reinforced on a regular basis. The committee might also consider having an annual open meeting so that interested professionals could attend and observe the committee in action. (This can be a valuable way to generate interest in becoming a potential member.)

The scope and sequence of ethics education for professionals should be similar to that of the biomedical ethics committee itself. The intensity and depth, however, will be to a much lesser degree. In general, professionals should be provided with definitions of ethical terms, background information about ethical theory and the biomedical ethics movement, and a description of cases that have had an impact on the medical profession. One of the most important components of ethics education for professionals, as well as for the committee, is the need to be kept aware of any factors that are currently being discussed in the field of ethics or any pending changes that may affect the health care delivery system.

Obviously, it would be impossible to provide all members of the professional staff with all the information being produced in the field of biomedical ethics. It is possible, however, to guide individuals to resources that contain more in-depth information on particular topics that they are interested in. Ethics books and articles available in the hospital library and notices posted about future ethics conferences can encourage independent research and continued involvement with a given topic. In some cases, distribution of up-to-date or crucial information will enhance committee visibility and credibility with other members of the professional staff.

Ethics Education for the Nonprofessional Staff

Ethics education within an institution should also reach nonprofessional staff members. In this book, *nonprofessionals* refer to those who do not usually have direct patient contact (such as workers in the business or medical records offices) or see patients in a nonclinical capacity (such as dietary workers or housekeeping staff). Although there are advantages to providing ethics education for the nonprofessional staff, educators should be aware of obstacles and limitations.

Advantages

It is probably accurate to say that the main focus of ethics education should be directed to the professional staff. However, there are several advantages to expanding these endeavors to include all interested hospital workers.

First, in today's health care climate, a great deal of emphasis is placed on the team effort required to provide comprehensive, high-quality, compassionate care to patients and their families. Everyone who works in a health care facility is part of the same team with the same mission and goals. By including all workers in ethics (and other) educational opportunities, an institution helps reinforce the value of each team member and assists in breaking down any territorial barriers that might exist. A team effort in health care can succeed only if all the people on that team have an awareness, and ideally an understanding, of the role they each play and of the many elements that go into the provision of comprehensive care.

A second reason to include the nonprofessional staff in ethics education is to inform them about what to do if they become aware of an on-the-job problem or ethical situation. Although nonprofessionals infrequently encounter such situations, ethics education will enable them to recognize and report problems should they occur. For example, a housekeeper may be alone in a room with a patient who comments that he does not really understand the purpose of his surgery. A maintenance staff person, while changing a light bulb, could find a patient's daughter in distress because she is afraid that her father is suffering unnecessary pain. A nonprofessional would not be expected to address these situations directly. However, there should be an expectation that the staff members would not ignore these events but would know that these comments need to be referred for appropriate follow-up as well as the correct process to make such a referral.

A final reason to provide ethics education to the nonprofessional staff is to enable them to have a better understanding of ethical issues and conflicts that they may encounter in their personal lives. Information learned and assimilated in the work setting can be transferred to family and community experiences. Many developments, conflicts, and court decisions are mentioned in the mass media and discussed outside health care settings. By providing a knowledge base to a variety of individuals, the health care institution assists in the dissemination of accurate, timely, and comprehensive information beyond the institutional walls. Individuals who have had experience with ethics education usually are better able to ask appropriate questions and make informed choices should the need arise for the provision of health care for a family member or loved one.

Obstacles and Limitations

There will, of course, be some hurdles and problems in efforts to include nonprofessional staff in ethics education. First, the nonprofessional staff will have neither a medical knowledge base nor a clinical background. Therefore, in addition to learning terminology related specifically to ethics, these individuals may need to learn many of the more standard medical terms.

Another obstacle to overcome is that nonprofessionals who feel that they have a limited clinical knowledge base may ask too many questions or, conversely, may be too intimidated to ask any questions at all. Ethics committees that are serious about providing ethics education to everyone would be wise to consider developing a series of preliminary programs targeted at providing a baseline for specific audiences before they integrate all employees into institutionwide ethics events.

The great intellectual diversity within the staff of any institution is another challenge to providing ethics education for everyone. Individuals who plan educational events and develop educational materials must remember to provide resources that are suitable for various intellectual levels and learning needs.

Additionally, confidentiality is a concern that may surface in a discussion of whether to include nonprofessionals in ethics education. There may be some apprehension that people who do not deal with confidential issues on a regular basis might inadvertently divulge privileged information. Although it is natural in the course of ethical discussions for information to be shared about specific cases, it is also expected that patients will not be identified by name. However, there is always the possibility that a patient's identity could become known. A review of the expectations for confidentiality at the beginning of each ethics presentation or discussion and regular reinforcement of these expectations should minimize breaches of confidentiality among all participants.

Perhaps the most difficult obstacle to overcome in the effort to include nonprofessionals in ethics education is the preconceived notion (usually held by members of the professional staff) that education on topics such as ethics should be reserved for "high-level" health care providers. Professional staff may feel that the presence of nonprofessionals would raise conflicts, create confusion, and ultimately encourage challenges to authority. It is the obligation of the ethics committee, therefore, to establish a framework that identifies the value of a more global and integrated approach to ethics education and to support the inclusion of the entire health care team in the process.

Integration of Biomedical Ethics Education into Other Institutional Activities

Although biomedical ethics can be approached as a specific educational program or series of events, the *application* of biomedical ethics theory, principles, and thinking cannot be isolated from the rest of the practice of medicine. Indeed, ethics and ethical reflection are intertwined in everything that happens in a health care setting. As such, it is important to encourage the conscious inclusion of a component of ethical awareness in a wide variety of institutional activities. These activities include:

- Orientation
- Departmental meetings
- One-on-one meetings
- Staff support groups
- Educational opportunities

Orientation

As new employees join the staff of a health care facility, it is important for them to be introduced to the concept of biomedical ethics, to the scope of biomedical ethics activities within the institution, or to both. They should be made aware of the role and function of the biomedical ethics committee, the policies that address ethical issues, and the type and scope of ethics-related educational opportunities that are available. New staff members should also be made aware of *their* expected role in ethics issues as well as the appropriate process to address ethical questions or concerns.

Departmental Meetings

A regularly scheduled departmental meeting can provide an ideal forum for individuals in similar job situations to discuss ethical issues in general or to review particular ethical questions and issues related to patients or on-the-job events that they have encountered. Directors and managers who encourage this type of discussion and allow time for it during staff meetings demonstrate the importance of the ethical component of health care, ultimately encouraging their staff members to be actively involved in the process of ethical thinking.

One-on-One Meetings

Some people are uncomfortable discussing difficult situations or controversial cases in a group setting. For these employees, individual meetings and one-on-one sessions to address specific concerns may be helpful and necessary.

In addition, many annual job performance evaluations include a section on mission or values. Any questions concerning the ethics process or the application of ethical theory can be addressed during this component of the evaluation discussion.

Staff Support Groups

Peer groups, established to support staff who work in units such as critical care, trauma/emergency, and neonatal intensive care, will most likely address ethical issues in the course of their discussions. Group members may not, however, name the ethical issues as such and may need to consciously identify the various ethical components and conflicts that affect their perceptions of their jobs and the services they provide. These groups will assist staff members in clarifying and coming to terms with difficult issues.

Educational Opportunities

Perhaps the most obvious, yet easily overlooked, opportunity to include ethics as a specific component of a certain topic, is in the content of the various educational programs held in health care institutions. During CME programs for physicians, nursing education events, general staff in-service programs, and conferences or seminars, ethics can be included along with topic-specific medical and patient care information. For example, discussions of the latest cancer treatments, updates on geriatric care, introductions of new medicines, and debates on health care reform issues can all include information concerning ethics and the ethical application of the information being presented. The key to the appropriate inclusion of an ethics component in this type of program is to discuss the application of these facts in relation to real situations.

Extension of Biomedical Education to the Community

The final phase of ethics education is to provide educational opportunities to the general community. Lay audiences are exposed almost daily to information in the mass media about situations, cases, and legal decisions that have an ethical dimension. The general community has an interest in, and a need to be informed about, the issues that are important to them, their families, their neighbors, and the world. Programs can be planned to educate lay audiences about advance directives and living wills, new medical technology, lifesaving measures such as cardiopulmonary resuscitation (CPR) or ventilators, and a host of other subjects that will enable individuals to understand their options and learn how to make informed health care choices.

Health care institutions can be proactive in their educational efforts by surveying their community to discover local topics of interest and designing events to address those needs. Information can also be provided to community members via literature, videos, or handouts. These resources may cover a variety of topics and may guide individuals to other sources, where they can obtain more information.

In the long run, an institution that develops a systematic method for identifying the needs of the community and then designs a comprehensive program that includes ethics information and a process for community members to address ethical questions will help eliminate health care conflicts before they arise.

Summary

Biomedical ethics education is a broad, extensive, and sometimes exhaustive multidimensional process. For it to be meaningful, it must be comprehensive as well as systematically planned and carefully executed. Individuals from all health care disciplines and from the general community can benefit from knowledge of ethics as a philosophical subject and from learning information that they can use as they apply ethical theory in practical situations.

Ethics education, done well, takes considerable time. It covers numerous topics that are continually changing. A plan for an ethics education program needs to combine fact, process, and theory in such a way that members of an interdisciplinary audience will be able to grasp the relationship between the knowledge that they have learned and the role that they play as part of the health care team.

References

1. Annas, G. J. Ethics committees: from ethical conflict to ethical cover. *Hastings Center Report* 21(3):29–32, May–June 1991.

2. Carms, A., editor. Forming an ethics committee: make no mistake about it. *Medical Ethics Advisor* 8(7):73–84, July 1992.

3. Ross, J. W. *Handbook for Hospital Ethics Committees*. Chicago: American Hospital Publishing, 1986.

4. Mappes, T. A., and Zembaty, J. S. *Biomedical Ethics*. 3rd ed. New York City: McGraw-Hill, 1991.

5. Solomon, M. Z., Jennings, B., Guilfoy, V., Jackson, R., O'Donnell, L., Wolf, S. M., Nolan, K., Koch-Weser, D., and Donnelley, S. Toward an expanded version of clinical ethics education: from the individual to the institution. *Kennedy Institute of Ethics Journal* 1(3):225–45, Sept. 1991.

Suggested Readings

Haddah, A. M. A source of support: an ethics committee helps nurses do the right thing. *Health Progress* 72(1):60–63, Jan.–Feb. 1991.

Iserson, K. V. Strategic planning for bioethics committees and networks. *HEC Forum* 3(3):117–27, 1991.

Jonsen, A. R. Of balloons and bicycles or the relationship between ethical theory and practical judgement. *Hastings Center Report* 21(5):14–16, Sept.–Oct. 1991.

Middleton, C. Institutional ethics committees. *Ethics, Sponsorship, and Pastoral Ministry* 1(3):1–7, Summer 1992.

Thompson, D. Hospital ethics. *Cambridge Quarterly of Healthcare Ethics* 3(3):203–15, 1992.

Chapter Three

An Overview of Biomedical Ethics Topics

The status of biomedical ethics today can be clearly understood only when examined in the context of the changes that have occurred in this field over the last several decades. The changing role of the patient, developments in medicine and technology, and shifts in the social and human condition have combined to create a complex core of theory and practice from which modern biomedical ethics has evolved.

One challenge of biomedical ethics educators is to give program participants sufficient information about historical developments in biomedical ethics. Understanding the past helps enrich and guide present ethics discussions and decision making. This chapter presents a general overview of the past and then provides an introduction to many of the most significant topics in biomedical ethics. It is *not* intended to cover all aspects of every biomedical ethics issue, but it does offer a synopsis of some of the most frequently discussed topics and areas in which conflicts often occur.

The Changing Role of the Patient

Modern medical ethics has been transformed and refocused by the reemergence of the *patient* as the primary force in the health care decision-making process. In recent years, there has been a noticeable and pervasive switch of emphasis away from the physician as primary decision maker and toward the patient as the one responsible for health care choices. The patient, who for a long time assumed a passive role in this process, is now not only assuming but demanding a more active role. As health care consumers, patients are becoming educated about their options and expressing their needs and desires.

In the early years of formalized medicine, the individual patient was always the primary focus of the physician. During the time of Hippocrates, disease was thought to be the result of an imbalance in the four humors of the body, and symptoms were treated in an attempt to bring these humors back into proper balance. Because each person was different from everyone else, the treatments used to regain this alignment were individualized for each patient.[1]

As medical knowledge advanced and specific disease entities were identified, physicians began to focus on the illness rather than on the patient who had the illness. Physicians began to approach care from a more scientific perspective and to search for patterns in illnesses that could be grouped and treated similarly. As the medical profession began to look at how diseased patients were alike, rather than on how they were different, the focus on the individual patient became diluted.

A second development that took the focus away from the individual patient was the advent of modern diagnostic procedures and technologies. In early medicine, physicians depended on the patient or on the patient's family to provide an anecdotal account of a medical problem. With the arrival of X-ray technology, laboratories, and advanced medical equipment, physicians no longer had to rely on observations and verbal reports but could call on scientific and objective data to provide necessary diagnostic information.

As the trend of medical advancement continued into the 20th century, treatment moved further away from being centered on the needs of the individual patient and more into the realm of physician prerogative. In the 1950s and 1960s, however, the pendulum began to swing back the other way. Although major medical and technological advances were occurring, this was a time when modern ethical and philosophical inquiry began, and the metamorphosis in modern medical ethics started to take hold. Society began to examine principle-based moral theories and patients began a movement to take back some measure of control in their health care.[2]

During this period, medical advances generated a number of situations that rendered inadequate the old ways of looking at these situations and making decisions about them. For example, for the first time in history, an individual could be kept alive through the use of an artificial respirator. In some cases, this technology was nothing short of a miracle. In other cases, the patient was kept alive, but in such a state that there was little or no hope of recovery. As a result, the quality of life of such patients was often seriously questioned.

Another example was that the artificial kidney could now be used to treat chronic kidney disease. However, there were not enough machines or funds to provide the service for all the people who needed the treatment. Certain questions arose. Who would get the service? What would be the selection criteria? Should the treatments be provided only to those who could afford them? Was not the indigent person just as worthy of care? Who would decide? When kidney transplants eventually became available, the same questions needed to be revisited.

Later, additional events brought the rights of patients to the forefront of discussions. These events included the U.S. Surgeon General's 1966 ruling that boards of review should be created at institutions conducting research on human subjects. This prevented arbitrary research without patients having a full understanding of the nature of the research in which they were involved. Another event was the development of consent forms to ensure that patients were made aware of the risks and benefits of any medical procedures they underwent and that they granted permission for the treatment or research procedures to take place. Other events that helped the patient rights movement include the 1973 *Roe v. Wade* U.S. Supreme Court decision stating that a woman has a legal right to have an abortion, and the development in the 1970s of the Patient's Bill of Rights, which, for the first time, informed hospitalized patients about the specific rights and information to which they were entitled.

As these changes occurred and the expectation of more advances began to be the norm, many individuals started looking seriously at how health care options and technological advances might affect them and their families. Many individuals began to fear that physicians would employ medical technology to extend their existence far beyond the point at which they believed there was any meaningful quality of life. They feared that decisions would be made *for* them that did not reflect their personal desires. It was at this point that many health care facilities, patients, and the legal community decided to become active in developing formal processes that would enable patients to state what they wanted or did not want in their medical care.

Many patients are now more concerned about their options, more aware of their rights, and more cognizant of personal responsibility for their own health care. The medical community, for the most part, has recognized this as a positive change and has taken steps to support and encourage the trend.

The Process of Patient Choice

The ongoing process of formalizing patient choices includes informed consent and documentation of choices. The following sections discuss these issues in more detail.

Informed Consent

The effort within the medical community to formalize a process that allows patients to have a voice in their medical care first began to take shape under what is commonly referred to as the *doctrine of informed consent.* This doctrine is accepted today by physicians, lawyers, ethicists, and others in health care, as the norm that should guide decision making in the context of a physician–patient relationship.

The doctrine of informed consent requires the following:[3]

1. Physicians must provide their patients with sufficient information about any proposed medical intervention so that each patient is aware of all aspects of that option and of the available alternatives.
2. Physicians must help patients understand information so that risks and benefits are clear and so that patients can make decisions consistent with their personal beliefs and values.

3. Physicians must be certain that the decision to accept or reject an intervention is the free and voluntary choice of the patient.

The doctrine of informed consent stresses the value of the autonomy of the patient, yet acknowledges that a decision-making process must be a collaborative effort.

On the surface, the doctrine of informed consent appears clear and easy to apply. However, this is not always the case. Although the doctrine requires that each patient have the option to accept, continue, reject, or discontinue an intervention, sometimes problems arise. For example, patients are not always capable of understanding the information presented to them. How can an informed decision be made when the patient is not able to cognitively process information about options?

In some cases, there may even be a question of whether to tell a patient about a specific diagnosis (for example, in a patient with suspected Alzheimer's disease). Unlike a patient with another type of chronic disease, such as cancer, a patient with symptoms of Alzheimer's disease cannot yet be given a definitive clinical diagnosis.[4] Does telling a patient with indications of early dementia that he or she may have Alzheimer's disease add to the patient's problems by increasing fear, perhaps ultimately decreasing patient involvement with his or her care? Is it then ethical—in light of the doctrine of informed consent—to withhold this information to maximize the patient's potential? At times, the application of the doctrine of informed consent becomes a matter of the *degree* to which the doctrine can be applied, rather than the duty to apply it.

Another type of problem arises when an individual requests a particular intervention that the physician believes will be of no medical benefit. The patient may be well informed and be aware of all of the possible consequences, yet may be very ill and therefore beyond the stage at which the requested treatment will be of any clinical value. How can such patient requests be balanced with the opinion, judgment, and conviction of the physician? Is it ethical to expend health care dollars for an "informed" patient who knows and accepts the risk, even though there is limited or no medical benefit? There are no easy answers.

Probably one of the most difficult aspects of helping patients to reach a reasonable, informed decision is that many such decisions have their roots in emotion. Patients often make choices based on perceptions rather than on a well-calculated analysis of the benefits, burdens, costs, and risks of every possible option. Patients tend to base decisions partly on past experience and (sometimes faulty) memories of a prior event or on anecdotal accounts and stories from other people who were in similar situations. They may also base decisions on irrational fears or unrealistic expectations of outcomes and on self-predicted short-term and long-term feelings. A decision may even be reached based on how the information was framed. Patients may perceive a 30 percent failure rate as being vastly different from a 70 percent success rate. Therefore, physicians, in applying the doctrine of informed consent, have an obligation to provide patients with guidance not only in the actual clinical decision-making process but also in the subjective analysis of perceptions that may affect their judgments.[5]

Physicians have a clear ethical obligation—and a legal requirement—to apply the doctrine of informed consent as broadly and as thoroughly as possible. Gone are the days when it was common practice for physicians and family members to make a decision to "protect the patient from the truth." Now, physicians and patients are obliged to work together to understand the specific disease or condition and to plan the course of future treatment.

Because of advances in knowledge and technology, the specifics of exactly how the doctrine of informed consent should be applied are still evolving. However, the doctrine has provided the basic foundation for the modern view of patient involvement in the health care decision-making process. As such, the doctrine of informed consent will remain a basic tenet on which future health care decisions are made.

Documentation of Patient Choice

For full compliance with the doctrine of informed consent, it is not sufficient to merely involve the patient in any decision-making process. It is necessary to document those choices to ensure that they will be carried out. Several methods have been developed that attempt to accomplish this task. These methods include:

- Consent forms
- Provisions of the Patient Self-Determination Act (PSDA)
- Advance directives

These methods are discussed in further detail in the following subsections.

Consent Forms

The first, and probably most familiar of these methods, is the *consent for treatment form*. This form has been in use for many years. It is used to verify that the patient has been given information about a treatment or procedure, that the risks and benefits have been explained, and that the patient has given permission for the event to take place. This form is used for a patient who is competent when the treatment or procedure will be performed relatively soon. A consent form is designed so that the physician can review it with the patient. The patient then signs and dates the document, which subsequently becomes part of his or her medical record.

Provisions of the Patient Self-Determination Act

Besides the need to verify a patient's agreement for impending procedures and treatments, it has become important to provide methods for documentation of choices about end-of-life decisions. In 1990, the federal government took a major step toward accomplishing this task by passing the Patient Self-Determination Act (PSDA). This act, which marks the first time that Congress has passed legislation concerning the ethics of life-sustaining treatment,[6] is a significant step toward the specific recognition of individual rights at the end of life. The act is designed to facilitate communication between the patient, the physician, other professional caregivers, and family members.

The act requires that health care facilities do the following:[7]

- Provide written information to each newly admitted patient concerning:
  - The patient's right to make decisions concerning medical care, including the right to accept or refuse medical or surgical treatment and the right to formulate advance directives
  - The policies of the organization that address the implementation of these rights
- Document in the patient record whether the individual has an advance directive
- Neither discriminate nor condition the provision of care, based on whether the patient has an advance directive (the act *does not require* individuals to complete an advance directive)
- Ensure compliance with state law in respect to advance directives
- Provide for education of staff and community concerning advance directives

The PSDA was not intended to answer all of the possible questions that might arise in relation to end-of-life decisions. It assumes, however, that if patients are informed of their rights, they will be more likely to take advantage of them. It also assumes that people who are actively involved in their health care decisions will be more likely to get the care that they believe is appropriate to their needs.

Advance Directives

An advance directive is different from an informed consent in that an informed consent is made by an adult capable of making a choice concerning *imminent* treatment, whereas an advance directive expresses health care decisions that an individual wants carried out at some unknown *future* date when that person is no longer capable of making a contemporaneous decision.

There are two major misconceptions about advance directives. One is that there is a perfect or correct form to use to document patient choice, and the other is that all advance directives must be written.[8] The desire to produce a perfect document arises from the need for clarification, in order to prevent any ambiguity in the future. Such a document would be clear in every circumstance, contain no areas that might be open to interpretation, and allow no room for questions. Although such a document would enable health care providers to approach their tasks with a high degree of certainty, in reality such a complex and intricate document would be impossible to design.

With regard to the second misconception, it is not true that an advance directive must always be written. Although a written document is preferable, oral statements concerning treatment preferences have been accepted when witnesses have been able to provide clear and convincing evidence concerning a patient's wishes.

When an advance directive is written, it provides a relatively clear picture of the patient's desires and also shows that the patient was serious about making his or her choices known. An oral advance directive, however, tends to be less detailed and less concrete. It is also open to interpretation by the individual to whom the information was given as well as by others involved in the patient's care.

Although the PSDA has been in effect since 1990, many individuals have not prepared an advance directive. The reasons for this include the following:[9]

- It is not clear who is primarily responsible for approaching the subject of advance directives. Physicians tend to see the responsibility as being patient centered. Patients, on the other hand, are not necessarily comfortable in taking on this task or in broaching the subject with their physicians.
- Some physicians are uncomfortable in talking with patients and family members about death or about end-of-life choices such as the withholding or withdrawal of treatment. Physicians have been trained to cure and to heal. The idea of making a conscious choice either not to start or to stop treatment may trouble some physicians. Some physicians believe that if they discuss these types of decisions, patients may become discouraged and react poorly to what they perceive as negative information, and that this will ultimately affect their prognosis.
- Unlike a century ago, when people died at a much younger age, most often at home, where a "death watch" was common, today many people in the younger generation have never experienced the loss of a family member. They and their physicians may view advance directives as being appropriate for the elderly or infirm, but unnecessary for the young and healthy. Consequently the subject may never be discussed.

Advance directives provide a valuable tool for physicians and health care providers to use in determining the end-of-life wishes of a particular patient. Once someone prepares an advance directive, it is expected that his or her caregivers will interpret and implement the directive in good faith.

There are instances, however, when there may be some uncertainty as to how closely a person would want an advance directive followed. For example:[10]

- A patient may have executed an advance directive several years before becoming incapacitated. In the interim, there may have been a significant medical advancement of which the patient was unaware. Might the knowledge of this advancement have altered this person's thinking in regard to the application of the new technology?
- A patient may have indicated choices on a written advance directive that are clearly contradictory to his or her known values, beliefs, and previously stated preferences. Family members and caregivers may question whether the patient wrote what was actually intended or whether there perhaps was some misunderstanding concerning the information from which the patient was making choices.
- A patient may have provided information that would support the withdrawal of life-sustaining measures. If, however, the physician believes that the family would be better able to accept the patient's death if a treatment that would briefly delay death were maintained a bit longer, then the withdrawal of such treatment may be delayed. In such cases, the physician often reports that the family is also being "treated" in addition to the patient.

Although advance directives may be challenged and reviewed by ethics committees or the courts (such as in situations just described), physicians and institutional providers honor almost all advance directives as written.

There are two major types of advance directives: *instructive* and *proxy*. Each has been developed to serve a particular purpose, and each is used under somewhat different circumstances.

Instructive Advance Directives (Living Wills)

An instructive advance directive is usually called a *living will* or a *directive to the physician*. A living will can be executed by any adult and is generally viewed as a statement of a person's intention that when he or she reaches the end of life, no extraordinary means are to be used to prolong the dying process. A living will provides basic information that is intended to be used if a patient becomes terminally ill or injured. It provides direction for decision making but is usually nonspecific in regard to disease, condition, or circumstance.

A living will can be revoked or changed at any time by the individual who originated the directive. If a patient becomes comatose or otherwise unable to communicate with the physician, the directive remains in effect for the duration of the condition or until communication ability is restored.

It is important to note that, under the common definition of a living will, such a directive does *not* indicate a request for any act or omission that will deliberately end life. It simply allows for the unrestricted progression of the natural dying process.

Because most health care facilities provide life-sustaining treatment unless there is evidence that the patient would want otherwise, an instructive advance directive is useful in clarifying specific end-of-life requests. It falls short, however, of meeting all health care decision-making needs.

Specifically, almost all living will legislation and the forms used to document living wills address only situations where there is a terminal illness or an irreversible coma. They do not address all possible medical contingencies, nor the many other health care decisions that have nothing to do with end-of-life decisions or with the withholding or withdrawal of treatment. Another limitation of living wills is that there can be problems with the nonspecificity of the language used in their writing. Terms such as *imminent death, terminal,* and *life sustaining* are somewhat vague and may present problems when the living will is executed.[11] Therefore, it is difficult, if not impossible, for health care providers to know that their interpretation of a living will is exactly what the patient intended. In order for patients to address these problems, an alternative option is to use a proxy advance directive.

Proxy Advance Directive (Durable Power of Attorney)

In a proxy advance directive, a patient arranges for a *durable power of attorney for health care,* which legally designates another individual (agent) to make health care and treatment decisions for the patient should he or she become incapacitated. Once a durable power of attorney for health care has been executed, it remains in effect indefinitely unless the patient has specified an expiration date or revokes the document.

The agent, who is presumably a trusted family member, friend, or legal advisor, is called on to be the decision maker only after the patient is rendered incapable of decision making due to illness or accident. (A proxy advance directive does not take effect merely because a patient is old or eccentric or has a physical disability.) The agent is someone who knows and understands the patient's values and wishes and is able to make decisions congruent with those that the patient would make if he or she were able to do so.

As with living wills, individual states differ in their laws regarding durable power of attorney and proxy decision making. Some states have durable power of attorney laws that are general and make no mention of medical decisions. Other states authorize proxy decisions through acts of "natural death." Still others permit agents to make medical decisions, specifically including those concerning the withholding or withdrawal of treatment. Biomedical ethics educators should learn the laws pertaining to their jurisdiction before they undertake any educational effort concerning this topic.

It should be noted that not all proxy decision making occurs under the specific application of a legal advance directive. Historically, family members have been called on by physicians, courts, and other members of the health care community to make decisions for incompetent patients. The Quinlan ruling in 1976 established the legal precedent for this activity, by giving the patient's father the authority to make medical decisions on his daughter's behalf, without direct evidence that she would have appointed him to do so.[12]

Ethical Issues at the End of Life

It has been clearly established that patients have the right to make health care decisions and choices about their individual treatments. Many of the choices that they will need to make are related to options for treatment at the end of their lives. New technology and recent medical advances have made the number of choices greater and the range of choices significantly more complex. The next two sections of this chapter discuss two end-of-life issues in detail: medical futility and the right to die.

Medical Futility

Many decisions that have to be made at the end of a patient's life are based on whether treatments for the patient are determined to be medically futile. The concept of *medical futility* is somewhat hard to define and has different interpretations for individuals, depending on their values and belief systems. A procedure, such as dialysis for a permanently unconscious patient, may be considered futile by one individual but necessary by another. There is also a distinction between a treatment that may be physiologically futile and one that may be psychologically futile. A treatment that may not alter the medical outcome for a particular patient may give great comfort to a patient or a family who wants "everything done." In general, medically futile treatment is considered to be an intervention that either will not provide a known benefit to a patient or will not likely alter the outcome of the patient's condition or disease process.

The concept of medical futility is complex, in part because it is based on probability and possibility, not on certainty. It is not always possible to say, on scientific grounds, which treatments will be of benefit to which patients. Therefore, any discussion of medical futility must combine both factual (medical) and subjective (moral) judgments.

A question arises as to the obligations of the medical profession to provide medically futile treatments simply because a patient or surrogate requests them. What are the duties and obligations of physicians to provide interventions that have been shown to have limited or no potential value or have little likelihood of success? Some of these issues have been decided in the courts. In one notable case, that of Helga Wanglie, the judge allowed a woman's husband, acting as surrogate, to decide to maintain the patient on a ventilator even though physicians had determined that Mrs. Wanglie was permanently unconscious and was not benefiting from the mechanical intervention. The judge based this decision on a previous statement by the patient that, for religious reasons, she would want to be kept alive.[13]

With all patients for whom additional medical treatment would likely be medically futile, the physician has an obligation to inform the patient and the patient's family of the medical situation and to encourage discussion so that they can make appropriate, informed decisions. The benefits and burdens must be addressed, and the rationale for the determination of the futility must be explained.

At present, there is no standard medical guideline for the determination of futility, and no social structure or process for handling cases of patients for whom additional treatments are determined to be medically futile. Each case must therefore be addressed on an individual basis, and conflicts must be handled as they occur.

The Right to Die

Going hand in hand with cases of medical futility are those that address a patient's right to die. The right-to-die issue is the direct result of significant medical advances that enable the patient's life to be maintained artificially for long periods of time. The medical care and treatment provided throughout life are intended to ease the known process that ultimately will end in death. Left alone, without medical intervention, this life process may include a brief period of frailty, a loss of consciousness, or the experience of pain. By making use of medical technology, however, this period may be extended for a long time—sometimes decades—and may result in an experience that is wanted by neither the patient nor the patient's family.

Although the claim of a right to die seems to contradict the basic constitutional right to life and to self-preservation, the substantive due process clause of the 14th Amendment can be interpreted as a basis for the right to die.[14] As such, there is a framework for the acceptance of a constitutional right to die and justification for developing mechanisms that will protect that right.

The main goal stressed by proponents of the right-to-die movement is the need and desire for patients to experience a peaceful death—one that combines medical, personal, and social elements to ensure that the experience of death will be dignified.[15] This includes the need to maintain individual autonomy and the right to refuse medical intervention. In most cases, discussion concerning the right to die specifically addresses the withholding or withdrawal of life support or life-sustaining interventions.

The right-to-die issue changes focus, however, when the emphasis shifts from a patient's right to refuse medical treatment that *might* result in death (such as the right to refuse surgery) to the right to refuse care that *will* result in death (such as the right to refuse food or hydration). Who, then, has the right to die? Is the right conferred only on people who are terminally ill? What about the right as applied to patients who are not near death but who are severely physically incapacitated, yet mentally competent? Does the right to die support the argument for assisted suicide or euthanasia? These ethical questions are significant not only in relation to patients themselves but also in relation to surrogates and agents, who need to make choices on behalf of patients.

Some of the issues surrounding right-to-die arguments include:

- Patient status
- Chronic and degenerative illness
- Active euthanasia and physician-assisted suicide
- Life-sustaining therapy

Patient Status

It is important to view end-of-life and right-to-die issues in the context of the medical status of the patients for whom such issues are relevant. Decisions concerning withholding and withdrawal of treatment are considered for patients at various points along the continuum of care. They are considered for patients who are brain-dead, patients who are in a persistent vegetative state (PVS), and patients who are seriously ill or impaired. In each case, the criteria applied in the decision-making process, and the ethical questions that arise, are unique and need to be addressed as they relate to that particular condition.

Brain Death

Once an individual is dead there is no longer a question as to whether treatments or procedures should continue, and there are no ethical issues concerning ceasing the provision of medical services to that patient. There is, however, an ethical (and practical) issue concerning exactly when an individual should be determined to be dead. In the past, when one vital organ system stopped functioning, the others soon followed and a physician could determine with certainty that the patient was dead. In the 1960s, however, that determination became less clear with the use of cardiopulmonary resuscitation (CPR) and respirators, which were able to maintain heartbeat and breathing for severely brain-damaged patients who were no longer capable of maintaining these functions independently. At that point, the traditional definition of *death*—the permanent cessation of the functioning of an organism—no longer applied. Instead, a new definition emerged, which focused on cessation of brain activity alone.

Within the definition of *brain death* there are three subdivisions:

- Whole brain death
- Neocortical death
- Brain-stem death

Whole brain death is defined as the permanent, irreversible cessation of the functioning of all areas of the brain. This can be determined by specific bedside tests and neurological evaluations that verify the absence of brain wave activity.

Neocortical death is defined as a cessation of the functioning of the higher brain centers, specifically, the cerebral hemispheres, which impart uniquely human characteristics such as identity, awareness of self and environment, and the ability to enjoy and experience one's surroundings. By strict definition of neocortical brain death, anencephalic neonates and persons in a persistent vegetative state would be considered dead.

The third category of brain death is *brain-stem death.* A definition of brain-stem death requires that only brain-stem activity cease before a patient is declared dead. By this definition, the brain stem *only* is the critical region that defines life. The risk in use of this criterion is that, on rare occasions, a patient may maintain consciousness through the higher brain, yet be totally unable to move, communicate, breathe, or feel.[16]

The adoption of brain-death criteria has been a key factor in the movement to encourage organ and tissue donation. Once a person has sustained a permanent cessation of brain function, his or her organ systems may be able to be maintained artificially until such time as vital organs can be removed for transplantation in an effort to save the life of another individual. At present, because of the ethical dilemmas surrounding the use of neocortical or brain-stem definitions, the whole-brain definition of brain death is the criterion most frequently used in determining whether to remove a patient from machines that artificially maintain bodily functions but that are not maintaining life.

When a patient who is to be removed from life support has healthy organs, most state legislatures now require that the family be informed about options for organ donation.[17] It is critical to inform family members that even though there may be artificially maintained activity in a patient's heart, lungs, or other organ system, the patient from whom organs would be transplanted is clinically and irreversibly dead. (Issues regarding organ and tissue donation are discussed in more detail later in the chapter.)

Persistent Vegetative State (PVS)

Patients who are in a PVS present a more difficult ethical problem than do patients who have experienced brain death, and the issues of termination of treatment for these patients tend to be more controversial and complex. *Persistent vegetative state* generally is defined as a relatively stable condition in which someone who (usually) had been neurologically normal is rendered incapacitated either because of acute brain trauma or because he or she is in the terminal stage of a chronic, progressive, degenerative disorder.

The most difficult aspect of the PVS is to determine whether a patient is experiencing the condition. This dilemma exists for a number of reasons. The condition itself lacks clear, consistent, specific diagnostic criteria. Although there is some general agreement concerning the nature of a PVS, consensus on the exact definition is lacking. Consequently, there are no laboratory or other tests that can be used to confirm or refute the diagnosis. Additionally, bedside examinations to determine the presence of a PVS are subject to a wide range of clinical and observational variability. Finally, it is not possible to interpret the *consciousness* of another individual by observation alone. Conclusions concerning the level of consciousness of a patient are therefore open to subjective interpretation.[18] The diagnosis of PVS must be made over the course of time and requires a lengthy period of observation in which no change in the patient's status occurs.

Another aspect of the difficulty in making a definitive diagnosis of PVS is that different patients fall at different points along the continuum of apparent brain activity. The specific point along the continuum that would validate neocortical brain death has not yet been established.

Patients in a PVS often exhibit similar characteristics. They maintain some normal brain-stem function[19] and thus usually have spontaneous breathing, pulse, and circulation. They have normal wake and sleep cycles and have some reflexes, such as cough, gag, and pupillary reaction to light. They may move their eyes and limbs but do not have purposeful movement. Chewing, swallowing, and speaking are not possible.

Patients in a PVS have no apparent awareness of themselves or their environment and do not relate to others in any way. Facial expressions such as smiles or grimaces may occur, but these facial movements are thought to be random and not expressive of emotion.

Patients who are in a PVS can be and often are kept alive for many years. These patients usually develop severe contractures and may require a tracheostomy tube to prevent respiratory disease. Patients in a PVS must be tube fed and are incontinent.

Although, according to currently accepted definition, patients in a PVS are not dead, they do not appear to be living either. As a result, questions related to the appropriateness of various treatment options or termination of treatment are common. For example, does the continuation of medical care for patients in a PVS constitute extraordinary care? If there is no hope of recovery for these patients, should they receive antibiotics if pneumonia develops? If a patient previously prepared an advance directive indicating that he or she would not want to be maintained under these circumstances, at what point should the decision to withhold artificial food and hydration be considered? Should all patients in a PVS have a do-not-resuscitate order?

These questions have no clear answers. Some individuals believe that life, no matter how limited, should be maintained at all costs. Others believe that to continue treatment for patients in a PVS constitutes extraordinary care and that to subject these patients to medical interventions is futile and an insult to the patients' human dignity.

A number of court cases have concerned patients in a PVS (most notably Cruzan[20]). Nevertheless, situations concerning PVS patients must be addressed on an individual basis. The beliefs of the patient, the needs of the family, and the resources available must all be taken into consideration in the determination of an appropriate and acceptable course of action.

Chronic and Degenerative Illness

Possibly the most challenging and complex cases involving right-to-die issues concern patients who are neither brain dead nor in a PVS but who have chronic, progressive diseases such as Alzheimer's disease, Huntington's chorea, multiple sclerosis, or acquired immunodeficiency syndrome (AIDS), or other debilitating conditions, such as cerebral palsy or severe burns. Some patients in these situations have requested that treatment be stopped and that they be allowed to die.[21] Other patients have taken matters into their own hands by taking actions that have hastened their deaths.

Active Euthanasia and Physician-Assisted Suicide

The issue of the "right" of a nonterminally ill patient to die—and the role of the medical profession in that "right"—has opened up a whole new complex area of ethical discussion: active euthanasia and physician-assisted suicide. The subject of "death by choice" is one of the most controversial and hotly debated topics in all of modern medical ethics. Although it has long been accepted practice to allow terminally ill patients to die by not initiating or continuing medically futile treatment (passive euthanasia), the idea of providing assistance to facilitate and enable a death (active euthanasia/mercy killing) is a relatively recent component of open medical, political, legal, and public discussions.

Active euthanasia is a voluntary act that results in the deliberate termination of the life of an individual, the intent of which is to eliminate pain and suffering. The goal of active euthanasia is to hasten an inevitable death that would likely be slow and agonizing. Euthanasia stops a life that would otherwise have continued for some time.[22]

Physician-assisted suicide is the provision, by a physician, of the directions, means, and/or assistance for a person to terminate his or her own life. The purposeful ending of one's life has been highly publicized through the actions of Dr. Jack Kevorkian, who has helped a number of individuals take their own lives, and through the success of such books as Betty Rollin's *Last Wish,*[23] about her mother's choice to end her own life rather than continue living with terminal cancer, and Derek Humphrey's *Final Exit.*[24]

Although physician-assisted suicide and active euthanasia are uncomfortable topics for many people, the issue of death by choice has been in the public eye in a number of ways. In the Netherlands, euthanasia is technically a crime, but authorities do not prosecute physicians who assist patients to die, and many individuals openly plan the time of their death. The Dutch system has been examined in the United States. Although the proposals were defeated, legalization of death by choice has been on the ballot in Washington state and California. The Hemlock Society has reported that some physicians regularly practice active euthanasia but do not, for obvious reasons, publicize their activity.[25] Patients are increasingly aware of their medical options, and, besides choosing an option to forgo treatment, some are actively requesting actions that will enable them to die at the time they desire.

It is through discussions of active euthanasia and mercy killing that one of the "slippery slopes" of medical ethics comes to light. In active euthanasia, it is presumed that the individual seeking death has made the choice to take this course of action and that the individual therefore agrees with the consequences. A conflict, however, arises in the discussion of active euthanasia for patients who are not conscious or who are not capable of making such a choice for themselves. If active euthanasia were to be legalized, how should surrogates make choices for or against the action? What criteria should be adopted to address cases such as those for severely impaired neonates? What is to be done concerning severely mentally handicapped individuals? The answers are far from resolved, and the discussions are complex. These ethical questions and the dilemmas concerning active euthanasia and assisted suicide are vast and will undoubtedly be discussed far into the future.

Life-Sustaining Therapy

For patients and surrogates to make informed choices concerning end-of-life decisions, it is important for them to understand the scope of the medical treatments about which they may need to make these choices. There are, of course, a wide variety of treatment options and medical procedures that could be recommended for an individual, and each of these options should be discussed thoroughly and carefully before any decisions are made. There are three areas, however, that seem to generate many of the most problematic ethical questions:

- The use of CPR and advanced cardiac life support
- The use of ventilators
- The provision of artificial nutrition and hydration

CPR and Advanced Cardiac Life Support

Cardiopulmonary arrest is the sudden cessation of ventilation (breathing) and systemic profusion (blood circulation). Cardiopulmonary resuscitation is the provision of temporary ventilation and circulation through artificial means, until advanced cardiac life support (ACLS) can be provided. Cardiopulmonary resuscitation is most successful when it is provided for otherwise healthy patients who have suffered a cardiopulmonary arrest and when an individual who is trained in CPR observes the situation and begins the procedure immediately.[26] In other cases, such as those in which an individual is found sometime after the actual arrest, or when an individual has another condition, the success rate is lower.

Cardiopulmonary resuscitation and ACLS have the same basic goal as do other medical interventions. They are designed to restore health, to eliminate suffering, and to preserve life. However, CPR and ACLS have another unique attribute in that the primary goal of these procedures is to reverse clinical death. This may not always be in the patient's best interest, and it also may not always be what the patient wishes.

All individuals experience a cardiopulmonary arrest at death.[27] Does this mean that all patients should be given CPR or ACLS? Unlike other medical procedures, no physician order is needed to initiate CPR or ACLS. Under the theory of implied consent, it is presumed that all hospitalized patients would want the procedures unless a statement has been issued to the contrary. As a result, CPR or ACLS (commonly called a CODE) is provided for all patients unless there is a no-CODE or do-not-resuscitate (DNR) order written on the patient's chart.[28]

Although the decision not to initiate a CODE for a patient is difficult and depends largely on personal needs and values, there are many situations in which it can be predicted that CPR or ACLS would provide no clinical value and could consequently be termed a futile intervention. For example, in patients who have metastatic cancer or sepsis or who have suffered a severe stroke, the provision of CPR or ACLS might serve only to prolong death, not prevent it. Also, when a patient is in a PVS, the provision of resuscitation cannot return the patient to normal cerebral function. Therefore, any resuscitation procedures performed on these patients could be considered futile.

The decision to provide or forgo resuscitation must be constantly evaluated and readdressed as a patient's condition changes. Because the perception of futility may vary over time, the CODE status of any patient should be constantly reviewed.

Through the PSDA, patients are entitled to state their wishes concerning the provision of CPR and ACLS. However, CODE status is a difficult subject to discuss with a patient, and it becomes harder to address as the patient becomes more ill. The patient and the family members may see this discussion as signaling that the physician has given up on the patient and may believe that a no-CODE order means no care. It must be made clear that no-CODE means only no resuscitation and that other treatments, such as antibiotics, transfusions, nutrition and hydration, and comfort care, may still be given. These other treatments are separate issues that will be dealt with independently from CODE issues.

A separate problem with a no-CODE order is that as a patient's condition deteriorates and surrogates assume decision-making power, the patient's wishes concerning a CODE may not be followed, especially if the patient's family states that they want "everything done." As a result, in some cases the staff may perform "slow CODEs" or "Hollywood CODEs" (half-hearted attempts at resuscitation). These CODES allow the patient to die, yet give the appearance of an attempt to continue treatment. The value and morality of these types of CODEs are topics of serious ethical debate.

In evaluating the decision to provide or withhold resuscitation, health care providers must review each case on an individual basis to determine whether resuscitation would meet a clear and specific clinical goal. When a goal is unlikely to be obtainable, a decision to withhold the treatment may be appropriate.

Mechanical Ventilation

When patients experience sustained respiratory failure (such as at the end stages of a chronic respiratory disease) as the result of neurological trauma, or after

CPR and are unable to breathe on their own, mechanical ventilation may be used to artificially maintain the actions of the lungs. Mechanical ventilation may be a temporary intervention, which is used only until the patient is again able to breathe independently, or it may become permanently necessary if a patient becomes physiologically dependent on the ventilator and is unable to be weaned off it.

Ethical issues arise concerning keeping patients on ventilators indefinitely. The idea of disconnecting a ventilator has serious implications for many individuals, and the decision to remove a patient from a ventilator is one that causes significant discussion among health care professionals and in ethics committees. This is especially true when a mentally alert and competent patient requests that he or she be removed from mechanical ventilation with the full understanding that such an action will result in death.[29] In these cases, careful psychiatric evaluation to determine the patient's mental status and a thorough review to clarify the patient's understanding of the situation are necessary before any action is undertaken. Mentally competent patients, however, *do* have the legal right to refuse medical treatment—even if that refusal will result in death.

For patients who are in a PVS or who are not competent, their previously stated desires, their prognosis, the length of time they have received mechanical ventilation, and other additional medical conditions must all be taken into account in determining the ultimate benefit or burden to the patient in relation to the continued use or withdrawal of mechanical ventilation. Because mechanical ventilation maintains life artificially, the removal of a patient from the machine does not *cause* death. Death is caused by the underlying pathology, which created the initial respiratory failure, and removal of a patient from a machine allows death to occur naturally.

Artificial Nutrition and Hydration

As with all potential treatments and medical interventions, the provision of artificial nutrition and hydration is appropriate when there is a potential benefit to the patient, when it is in accord with the patient's wishes, and when no harm will be done to the patient. This particular intervention, however, is somewhat different from others in that the very act of providing food and water is basic to all human interaction and relationships. This is true across time, race, religion, and culture and consequently is highly symbolic of love, loyalty, compassion, and concern. The thought of *not* providing nutrition and hydration raises many value-laden issues related to abandonment and rejection, which may have little to do with medical intervention or care.

As a patient approaches death, tolerance for oral acceptance of food and water naturally diminishes. As a result, family members are usually willing to agree that the provision of artificial food and hydration at this point would serve no beneficial purpose and that the initiation of tube feedings or the continuation of artificial feeding would only prolong the dying process. The issue of the appropriateness of providing artificial food and hydration is less clear, however, for patients who are in a PVS or coma or who are otherwise disabled but not terminally ill.[30]

As with other life-sustaining treatments, the decision to provide or forgo artificial food and hydration not only needs to be initially assessed for each patient but also needs to be reassessed on a regular basis. A decision to provide artificial nutrition and hydration can be changed to withhold the treatment if a later assessment indicates that the burden of treatment has begun to outweigh the benefits.[31]

Additional Ethical Issues

Although many ethical issues are related to death, dying, and end-of-life decisions, a significant number of issues that provide additional areas of ethical debate have emerged in recent years. These include genetic research and therapy, organ and tissue donation, issues involving the unborn, and allocation of resources.

Genetic Research and Therapy

Since the discovery in the 1950s of the structure and function of DNA, there has been an explosion of new developments in biomedical genetics, including the new sciences of gene therapy and genetic engineering. In the last several years, these topics have become matters of international curiosity and global ethical concern.

The most prominent activity in this field is the Human Genome Project. This massive effort has the goal of mapping, in detail, the position of all human genes on their respective chromosomes, in order to catalog the sequence and structure of each gene for human individuals. The entire project will identify more than 100,000 genes on the 46 human chromosomes and has the potential to alter our understanding of the total picture of human genetics.[32]

Information learned from the Human Genome Project will allow scientists and physicians to understand what normal human DNA should look like and may enable them to identify areas of abnormality within DNA. Scientists expect that, in the future, they may be able to correct abnormal areas of DNA through gene therapy.

There are two basic types of gene therapy: somatic cell therapy and germline alterations. In *somatic cell therapy* a defective gene is treated by replacing it with a normal one. At present, there are more than 4,000 identified genetic diseases involving a single defective gene. These diseases, such as sickle cell disease, Tay-Sachs disease, and cystic fibrosis, cause an estimated 7 percent of all neonatal deaths, affect approximately 1 percent of newborns, and are responsible for 10 percent of all childhood deaths. About half of these genetic diseases cause early death, and almost three-fourths of the rest produce debilitating impairments that are incompatible with normal life.[33] Clearly, these thousands of deaths and the huge medical costs involved in the care of patients with these diseases provide a rationale for determining ways to eliminate the genetic defects.

In the second type of gene therapy, *germ-line alterations*, an attempt is made to insert genetic changes into the reproductive cells of an individual, in order to change the set of genes passed on to a future generation. This type of gene therapy has a potentially high level of emotional impact and has opened significant ethical debate about the possibility for improper application. At issue are not only the prevention and identification of diseases and conditions but also the alteration and manipulation of a species. For example, if there is the capability of altering the species to produce healthy individuals, is there also the possibility of artificially producing enhancements[34] or alterations in physical attributes, such as height or eye color? Is there a possibility of producing offspring who have a high intelligence quotient or the ability to play the piano? Germ-line gene therapy—which exists only in theory at this point—has the potential to eliminate a great deal of pain and suffering. It also has the potential to alter the human race as we know it today.

No one knows the full impact that germ-line alterations or the Human Genome Project will ultimately have. It is known, however, that there may be vast medical, social, and political implications of genetic research and genetic services and that there will likely be far-reaching, long-range, ethical implications of any newly understood genetic knowledge.

Organ and Tissue Donation

Organ and tissue donation has become accepted in our society and is a relatively commonplace component of medical practice. When transplantation first became an option, the ethical issues were concerned with donations of kidneys and subsequently the heart. Now transplants are possible for lungs, liver, corneas, pancreas, and even bones. Modern technology is quickly approaching the capability to replace almost any organ in the body, and with this capability comes the awesome task of making an ethical determination of how to distribute the limited available organs to those in need.

Even though considerable media attention is given to the value and results of organ and tissue donation, the number of suitable donors who actually provide organs is relatively low. This is primarily due to the emotional factors surrounding organ donation. It is also difficult to approach families who have just experienced a tragedy and ask their permission to remove organs from a loved one for transplantation.

Organ and tissue donation may take place after an individual has been declared brain dead. The ethics of relaxing the definition of brain death to include persons in a PVS and anencephalic infants as a way to provide additional organs for transplantation has been discussed but remains unresolved.

Some of the other issues concerning transplantation of organs and tissue are related to equitability of distribution of resources, selection criteria for recipients, multiple sequential transplants for the same recipient, and the potential for organs to be bought and sold as commodities.[35]

There is some debate concerning the long-term value of organ and tissue transplantation. Does it really contribute to longevity, and does the cost–benefit ratio justify such major expenditures? As the capabilities of transplant technologies change, there will need to be continued debate concerning these and future ethical issues.

Issues Involving the Unborn

One of the most visible and controversial ethical issues in the United States is that of abortion. This issue illustrates perfectly the concept of ethical values in conflict. The abortion issue will most likely never be resolved regardless of any laws passed or cases decided in the courts.

One of the things that has added fuel to the debate over abortion is that over the last 20 years, the clinical status of the fetus has been altered by advances in medical technology. At one time, the fetus was considered to be a part of the mother. The fetus was not directly observable and could be assessed only indirectly. Now, through the use of high-resolution ultrasonography; sampling of fetal blood, tissue, and urine; and fetal monitoring, the fetus can be observed as a separate individual.

This maternal–fetal dyad, or the two-patient model,[36] presents a unique set of ethical issues that must be considered in the making of decisions about medical interventions. For example, in making health care choices, is it appropriate to look at the benefits versus burdens for the combination of the mother and the fetus or for each as individuals? Should fetal therapy, such as intrauterine surgery to correct an anomaly, be performed against the desire of the mother? What rights does a fetus have?

Some other issues involving the unborn are as follows:

- Is it ethically appropriate to use tissue from aborted fetuses for transplantation into another fetus to correct genetic diseases? (This could lead to abortions done specifically to obtain the needed cells.)
- Should children be conceived specifically to provide cells that can later be transplanted into an ill sibling?[37]
- Is it ethical to provide "womb rental" for surrogate parenting?
- What are the implications of selective termination of multiple embryos following multiple conception due to the use of fertility drugs?

Ethical issues involving the unborn have many legal, medical, and social implications and raise numerous questions. It is likely that these questions will integrate with new ones as technology continues to add new components to the prenatal ethics debate.

Allocation of Resources

Perhaps the most challenging, and certainly the most pervasive, issue about which there is ethical debate is the allocation of financial resources for medical care. As technology and medical capabilities have advanced and as populations have increased and aged, the need and desire for comprehensive medical care have grown far beyond the capability of providing it equitably to all. There continues to be ongoing discussion on the need for further reform of health care delivery systems and on the allocation of services to patients in need.

Relationships between patients, physicians, nurses, and other health care providers rest on certain ethical assumptions: adherence to standards, pursuit of knowledge, service to others, and a primary responsibility to provide services and care that are in the best interests of the patient. The bottom line in this model is an expectation that there will be the greatest good provided to the greatest number of people in the most cost-conscious but effective and high-quality manner possible. This makes sense in theory, but these qualities are difficult for health care providers to define and almost impossible to implement.

In the United States in particular, there is a strong belief in individual freedom and individual rights. The impact that this belief has on allocation of resources is far-reaching, and as reform of the health care system continues, these individual rights may need to become subordinate to the rights of the country as a whole.

The economic problems facing the health care field are immediate, serious, and fundamental. There is clearly an ethical obligation to eliminate waste in health care practices, but first there must be an understanding of where that waste exists. Because the definition of waste, as with other ethical issues, is subjective, agreement as to how to implement a waste-elimination process is under constant review.

As health care and technology advance in the future, choices will need to be made on a number of fronts. These choices will be made by patients, practitioners, institutions, and governments. Personal ethical responsibility will be a component of social justice, which will be weighed as part of the common good for present-day society and for the well-being of future generations.

Summary

Biomedical ethics covers a wide variety of topics and issues (some of which have been touched on here) that have been evolving and broadening over the last several decades. The role of the patient in the health care decision-making process is an important and prominent issue. Patient rights and the execution of those rights have become a major focus in the provision of medical and health care services. When informed consent is obtained, patient autonomy and the right to make personal choices are protected.

Through the passage of the PSDA and through the use of advance directives, living wills, and durable powers of attorney, it is now possible for patients not only to have a better understanding of the medical options being offered but also to make and document clear, conscious choices as to which of those options they believe are most desirable.

Many biomedical ethics issues involve decisions that must be made at the end of a patient's life. These decisions are concerned with questions of medical futility, a patient's right to die, or the withholding or withdrawal of treatments, such as CPR, mechanical ventilation, or artificial food and hydration. Biomedical ethics is also concerned with the ethical implications of genetic research, organ and tissue donation, procedures involving the unborn, and the allocation of health care resources.

As the field of medicine continues to evolve and as new technology provides patients, physicians, and health care workers with a wider variety of health care options, the field of biomedical ethics also will continue to evolve by incorporating these changes and providing a means to examine them in relation to ethical and moral principles.

References

1. Reiser, S. J. The era of the patient: using the experiences of illness in shaping the mission of health care. *JAMA* 269(8):1012–14, Feb. 24, 1993.
2. Pellegrino, E. D. The metamorphosis of medical ethics: a 30-year retrospective. *JAMA* 269(9):1158–62, Mar. 3, 1993.
3. deBlois, J. Ethical issues in health care: informed consent and the purpose of medicine. *Center for Health Care Ethics* 12(6):1–2, Feb. 1991.
4. Drickamer, M. A., and Lacks, M. Should patients with Alzheimer's disease be told their diagnosis? *New England Journal of Medicine* 362(14):947–51, Apr. 2, 1992.
5. Redelmeier, D. A., Rozin, P., and Kahneman, D. Understanding patients' decisions: cognitive and emotional perceptions. *JAMA* 270(1):72–76, July 7, 1993.
6. McCloskey, E. L. The Patient Self-Determination Act. *Kennedy Institute of Ethics Journal* 1(2):163–69, June 1991.
7. Hackworth, C. B., editor. New law requires hospitals to ask about living wills. *Medical Ethics Advisor* 7(1):1–8, Jan. 1991.
8. King, N. Dying made legal: new challenges for advance directives. *HEC Forum* 3(4):187–99, 1991.
9. LaPuma, J., Orentlicher, D., and Moss, R. Advance directives on admission: clinical implications and analysis of the Patient Self-Determination Act of 1990. *JAMA* 266(3):402–5, July 17, 1991.
10. Brock, D. W. Trumping advance directives. *Hastings Center Report* Special supplement:2–3, Sept.–Oct. 1991.

11. Sabatino, C. Durable power of attorney laws gaining some acceptance. *Medical Ethics Advisor* 6(8):105–9, Aug. 1990.

12. Emanuel, E., and Emanuel, L. Proxy decision making for incompetent patients. *JAMA* 267(15):2067–71, Apr. 15, 1992.

13. Troug, R. D., Brett, A. S., and Frader, J. The problem with futility. *New England Journal of Medicine* 326(23):1560–63, June 4, 1992.

14. Kass, L. R. Is there a right to die? *Hastings Center Report* 22(6):44–45, Nov.–Dec. 1992.

15. Callahan, D. Pursuing a peaceful death. *Hastings Center Report* 23(4):33–38, July–Aug. 1993.

16. Bernat, J. L. How much of the brain must die in brain death? *Journal of Clinical Ethics* 3(1):21–26, Spring 1992.

17. Sanders, L. M., and Raffin, T. A. The ethics of withholding and withdrawing critical care. *Cambridge Quarterly of Healthcare Ethics* 2(2):175–84, 1993.

18. Bernat, J. L. The boundaries of the persistent vegetative state. *The Journal of Clinical Ethics* 3(3):176–80, Fall 1992.

19. Hackworth, C. B., editor. Discrimination law clashes with bioethics over PVS. *Medical Ethics Advisor* 7(7):81–84, July 1991.

20. Phillips, D. F., editor. Cruzan ruling prompts individual and state actions. *Hospital Ethics* 6(5):1–5, Sept.–Oct. 1990.

21. Gibbs, N. Love and let die. *Time* 135(12):62–71, Mar. 19, 1990.

22. Loewy, E. H. Healing and killing, harming and not harming: physician participation in euthanasia and capital punishment. *Journal of Clinical Ethics* 3(1):29–34, Spring 1992.

23. Rollin, B. *Last Wish.* New York City: Linden Press/Simon & Schuster, 1985.

24. Humphrey, D. *Final Exit.* Eugene, OR: Hemlock Society, 1991.

25. Brodeur, D., editor. Physician assisted suicide: the debate of tomorrow, today. *Issues* 8(2):1–8, Mar.–Apr. 1993.

26. Neimann, J. Cardiopulmonary resuscitation. *New England Journal of Medicine* 327(15):1075–79, Oct. 8, 1992.

27. Lo, B. Understanding questions about DNR orders. *JAMA* 265(14):1874–5, Apr. 10, 1991.

28. American Medical Association, Council on Ethical and Judicial Affairs. Guidelines for the appropriate use of do-not-resuscitate orders. *JAMA* 265(14):1868–71, Apr. 10, 1991.

29. Edwards, M. J., and Tolle, S. Disconnecting a ventilator at the request of a patient who knows he will then die: the doctor's anguish. *Annals of Internal Medicine* 117(3):254–56, Aug. 1, 1992.

30. Grisez, G. Should nutrition and hydration be provided to permanently unconscious or otherwise mentally disabled persons? *Issues in Law and Medicine* 5(2):165–79, Fall 1989.

31. Koshuta, M. A., Schmitz, P. J., and Lynn, J. Development of an institutional policy on artificial hydration and nutrition. *Kennedy Institute of Ethics Journal* 1(2):133–40, June 1991.

32. Moraczewski, A. S., editor. Genes and ethics. *Ethics and Medics* 16(5):2–4, May 1991.

33. Munson, R., and Davis, L. H. Germ-line gene therapy and the medical imperative. *Kennedy Institute of Ethics Journal* 2(2):137–58, June 1992.

34. Fletcher, J. C., and Anderson, W. F. Germ-line gene therapy: a new stage of debate. *Law, Medicine and Health Care* 20(1–2):26–39, Spring–Summer 1992.

35. Thomasma, D. C. Ethical issues and transplant technology. *Cambridge Quarterly of Healthcare Ethics* 1(4):333–42, 1992.

36. Mattingly, S. S. The maternal-fetal dyad: exploring the two patient obstetrical model. *Hastings Center Report* 22(1):13–18, Jan.–Feb, 1992.

37. Morrow, L. When one body can save another. *Time* 137(24):54–58, June 17, 1991.

Suggested Readings

Chervenak, F. B., and McCullough, L. B. Justified limits on refusing intervention. *Hastings Center Report* 21(2):12–17, Mar.–Apr. 1991.

Emanuel, L. L., Berry, M. J., Stroeckel, J. D., Ettelson, L. M., and Emanuel, E. Advance directives for medical care: a case for greater use. *New England Journal of Medicine* 324(13):889–95, Mar. 28, 1991.

Friedman, E., editor. *Choices and Conflict: Explorations in Health Care Ethics*. Chicago: American Hospital Publishing, 1992.

Friedman, E., editor. *Making Choices: Ethics Issues for Health Care Professionals*. Chicago: American Hospital Publishing, 1986.

Jecker, N. S. Knowing when to stop: the limits of medicine. *Hastings Center Report* 21(3):5–8, May–June, 1991.

Jecker, N. S., and Schneiderman, L. J. Medical futility: the duty not to treat. *Cambridge Quarterly of Health Care Ethics* 2(2):151–59, 1993.

Jonsen, A. R. Beyond the physician's reference: the ethics of active euthanasia. *Western Journal of Medicine* 2(149):195–98, Aug. 1988.

Mason, D. On behalf of the patient. *Hastings Center Report* Special supplement:9–10, Sept.–Oct. 1991.

Meier, D. E. Physician assisted dying: theory and reality. *Journal of Clinical Ethics* 3(1):35–37, Spring 1992.

Miles, J. Protecting patient self-determination. *Health Progress* 72(3):26–30, Apr. 1991.

Miles, S. H. Medical futility. *Law, Medicine, and Health Care* 20(4):310–15, Winter 1992.

Ross, J. W. Judgements of futility: what should ethics committees be thinking about? *HEC Forum* 3(4):201–10, 1991.

Rouse, F. Patients, providers and the PSDA. *Hastings Center Report* Special supplement:2–3, Sept.–Oct. 1991.

Sulmasy, D. P., Geller, G., Faden, R., and Levine, D. The quality of mercy: caring for patients with do not resuscitate orders. *JAMA* 267(5):682–86, Feb. 5, 1992.

Chapter Four

A Process for Ethical Thinking and Reflection

It is both interesting and important to have an understanding of the historical, medical, social, and legal developments in the field of biomedical ethics. This knowledge, however, becomes truly useful only when it is applied to real situations involving actual patients and their families.

It is therefore essential for any biomedical ethics education plan to include periodic programs containing factual information as well as ongoing education on both a process and a standardized framework for applied ethical thinking and reflection. Familiarity with this kind of process enables health care workers to develop a comfort level with the kind of facts used in ethical reflection and with the steps that need to be taken to facilitate making an appropriate ethical decision.

A standardized process for ethical thinking and reflection is important in two key areas of a comprehensive biomedical ethics program. First, it provides a consistent set of guidelines and direction for members of the biomedical ethics committee as they conduct patient case consultations. Second, it provides an organized way of presenting situations and cases for discussion at educational events.

Although the components of a process for ethical thinking and reflection are basically the same in both applications, the depth to which the process is applied will vary depending on the setting. It can be expected that a biomedical ethics committee will tend to apply the process in great detail as it conducts a case consultation. (See figure 4-1.) However, during an educational program, which would likely be limited by time constraints, any one area of the process may be emphasized to a greater degree than another, and the content presented may be less detailed. (See figure 4-2.)

By establishing a standardized process for ethical thinking and reflection, an institution provides a framework for case analysis that is clear, logical, comprehensive, and easily documented, thus diminishing the risk of emotional, subjective, and unproductive debates on issues or cases. The remainder of this chapter presents one example of a possible model for a process for ethical thinking and reflection. Any institution that undertakes the task of providing ethics education would benefit from developing a similar model that contains components important to that institution's own philosophy and values.

Figure 4-1. Sample Guidelines for Ethical Thinking and Reflection, Case Consultation Form

Community Hospital
Hometown, PA 19000

Guidelines for Ethical Thinking and Reflection
Biomedical Ethics Committee
Case Consultation Form

Patient ____________________ M/F DOB ____________ Medical record # ________

Name/relationship of next of kin ____

Primary physician ____

Other physicians involved:

______________________________ ______________________________

______________________________ ______________________________

Date of consultation _______________ Time _______________ to _______________

Reason for request ____

____

Consultation participants: Patient? Yes/No

Biomedical ethics committee members:

______________________________ ______________________________

______________________________ ______________________________

______________________________ ______________________________

Others:

______________________________ ______________________________

______________________________ ______________________________

______________________________ ______________________________

Medical/treatment/care information:

Diagnosis/prognosis

Course of present illness/hospitalization

Treatment history

Activities of daily living

Other

Who are the interested parties and what is their involvement with this case?

Are there any legal/administrative concerns?

What are the ethical issues/conflicts?

What ethical principles are involved?

____ Autonomy ____ Beneficence/nonmaleficence ____ Justice

____ Other: ____

Figure 4-1. (Continued)

What is known about the patient's perspectives on the present situation?

Is there a living will or durable power of attorney? If so, what do they say?

Is there a surrogate/legal guardian? ____ Who? ____________________

What are the treatment options and the potential consequences of each?

What appears to be in the best interest of . . .

The patient:

The family/surrogate/guardian (and so on):

The physician/health care workers:

The institution/society:

Points of discussion and other pertinent information:

Committee recommendation:

Notification of recommendation:

Given to: By whom: Date:

____

____

____

Is this case recommended as a topic for grand rounds? ____

Consultation form completed by ____________________ Date ______

Figure 4-2. Sample Guidelines for Ethical Thinking and Reflection, Educational Program Form

Community Hospital
Hometown, PA 19000

Guidelines for Ethical Thinking and Reflections
Education Program
Retrospective Case Review Form

Date ______________

What were the facts?

Medical:

Interested parties:

Patient's level of competency:

Legal/administrative issues:

What were the unresolved issues/ethical conflicts?

What ethical principles are involved?

____ Autonomy ____ Beneficence/nonmaleficence ____ Justice

____ Other: ____

What were the patient's wishes?

What were the treatment options?

What was in the best interest of each of the involved parties?

How was the case resolved?

Other:

There are six basic steps in a process for ethical thinking and reflection. These are:

- Step 1. Gather the facts.
- Step 2. Develop an understanding of the concerns, issues, or ethical conflicts.
- Step 3. Clarify the patient's perspective.
- Step 4. Identify the treatment alternatives.
- Step 5. Determine what is in the best interest of all involved parties.
- Step 6. Select the most appropriate alternative.

This chapter discusses these steps in detail.

Step 1: Gather the Facts

The first step in the process is to find out the pertinent facts relating to all aspects of the case being discussed. Clear, concise presentation of these facts should provide a synopsis of the history as well as the present status of the patient. Pertinent information includes medical facts, information about interested parties, the patient's level of competency, and legal and administrative facts.

Medical Facts

Medical facts provide the foundation for any case being reviewed. The medical information should cover the entire spectrum of the patient's condition, so that reflection on the ethical issues can be based on a thorough analysis of the clinical situation.

Medical facts should include (but are not limited to):

- Age and gender of the patient
- Diagnosis
- Course of present illness
- History of treatments and results
- Present hospitalization
- Medications
- Other contributing conditions or disabilities
- Status of daily living skills (ambulation, feeding, hydration, communication, and so on)
- Possible treatments and potential outcomes
- Recommended medical course of action
- Prognosis and life expectancy

Good ethics comes from good facts. It should be noted that many medical facts, such as statements concerning prognosis, expectations of treatment outcomes, and life expectancy, are in actuality probability statements and that not all physicians or clinical experts would necessarily have the same opinion concerning these statements. When differences of opinion are evident, clinicians should be as clear as possible concerning the information on which their own clinical judgments have been based.[1]

Information about Interested Parties

After the medical facts are identified, it is important to provide information concerning the interested parties in the case. Obviously, the patient is the person who has the greatest interest. There may also be an individual (a surrogate) who has been designated to represent the patient if the patient is unable to provide his or her own information.

The list of possible individuals who may be considered interested parties can be extensive. Some of the possibilities include the following:

- Spouse
- Adult or minor children
- Legal guardian
- Surrogate/proxy
- Significant other
- Lawyer
- Minister, priest, rabbi, or other religious leader
- Friend
- Health care providers

In addition, there may be a number of other individuals who have an interest in the case and who may be concerned with ethical issues or conflicts. Because of confidentiality regulations, it may not be possible to include these individuals in specific discussions or in patient-centered case consultations, yet it may be helpful to have their input when ethical issues are being discussed. It is therefore important to determine the following:

- Who are the interested parties?
- What is the relationship of these individuals to the patient? To each other?
- How well do the individuals understand the medical situation and the patient's condition?
- What is each person's interest in the case, and do they stand to gain or lose anything through a certain course of action?
- What information have the individuals provided to help clarify the situation?
- Are there conflicts among these individuals or between any of them and the patient?

Some cases are complicated because there is *no one* who is an interested party. This can present a whole different set of ethical issues, and the institution must make arrangements to appropriately provide someone to represent the patient. If this is the situation, information concerning the provisions that have been made should be identified.

The Patient's Level of Competency

The actual and potential level of competency must be established for any patient about whom there is an ethical question or situation. It is important to know the level of competency to determine that patient's present decision-making capacity and his or her expected capacity in the future.

The level of competency for a particular patient at any given moment will fall somewhere along a continuum from fully competent (awake, oriented, stable, and aware) to totally incompetent (in a persistent vegetative state or an irreversible coma). Patients on either end of this continuum present a rather uncomplicated picture in terms of decision-making capacity. The fully competent individual has every right to make health care decisions that are in keeping with his or her own values, and as long as no laws are being broken, requests to provide or not provide specific treatments are usually honored. In the other extreme, a proxy decision maker or a court-appointed legal guardian can be retained for the patient who is totally incompetent, and that individual can then make decisions on behalf of the patient.

Problems tend to arise when a patient's competency level falls somewhere in the middle of the continuum. For example, a patient may be awake and interested in participating in decision making, yet may be somewhat confused and depressed. A patient may understand part of the medical information that has been presented, yet may be unsure of the implications for certain courses of treatment. Also, some patients may be quite capable on one day but very disoriented and inconsistent in their decisions on another day. In many cases, a psychological evaluation or a mental status examination may be useful in establishing facts concerning the level of competency of a patient.

Legal and Administrative Facts

Legal and administrative issues and other external factors, such as financial considerations, may have an impact on ethical considerations. It is therefore important to know whether similar situations have been addressed in the courts and whether there are any laws, statutes, or regulations that apply to the case. Any potential liability issues should be stated, and known legal precedents need to be identified and explained. In addition, hospital or institutional policies and procedures that apply need to be identified, and any applicable information from systemwide regulations (such as the Ethical and Religious Directives for Catholic Health Care Facilities) should be stated and clarified.

Finally, it is necessary to identify any important financial issues. The financial implications for the patient, the family, the institution, or society as a whole may influence any decisions.

Step 2: Develop an Understanding of the Concerns, Issues, or Ethical Conflicts

The need for case consultation or ethical review exists only when there is a concern about specific treatment, when there are unresolved issues, or when a conflict exists related to the appropriate course of medical care to be provided. These conflicts can be related to a particular patient or may exist when there are differences of opinion concerning a suggested course of action for a group of patients (for example, organ transplantation from anencephalic newborns).

An ethical conflict can arise between two or more of the interested parties and becomes a dilemma either when moral issues are involved or when there is conflict over the application of ethical principles. Conflicts relating to moral issues and conflicts of ethical principles are discussed in the following subsections. (It is important to remember that not all difficult situations arising in health care settings are due to ethical conflicts and would need to be reviewed by the process for ethical thinking and reflection. Many problems may be the result of other factors, such as poor communication, lack of medical knowledge, or emotional distress. In these situations, there is no ethical conflict, and the issue should be addressed through other resources at the facility.)

Conflicts Relating to Moral Issues

Moral issues become ethical conflicts when one or more individuals are asked to do something with which they disagree. These issues may be based in moral teachings of a particular religion, in cultural customs, or in a personal philosophy of what is right and wrong.

In general, the moral obligation in medicine and health care is to promote what is in the patient's best interest by using measures to benefit the sick, by taking steps to keep the patient from harm, and by preventing injustice.[2] An ethical dilemma arises when different individuals have diverse opinions concerning how these obligations are to be defined and how they are to be carried out. A dilemma is often created because a choice must be made between two (or more) possible correct or "good" courses of action. Specific identification of these choices, and of the conflicts that they create, is central to the process for ethical thinking and reflection.

Conflicts of Ethical Principles

The ethical principles about which conflicts and dilemmas frequently develop are:[3]

- Autonomy
- Beneficence and nonmaleficence
- Justice

Autonomy

The principle of autonomy refers to the right of all competent patients to make their own choices concerning health care and to decide on desired treatments of disease and illness. This principle is based on the belief and constitutional right that individuals should have control of their personal destiny in accordance with their own values and beliefs. In addition, even though these values and beliefs may be unique to each individual—and consequently may not be shared by others—as long as they are within the law and do not conflict with the standards of the institution, they should be honored, respected, and implemented.

The principle of autonomy has at its core the doctrine of informed consent. As discussed in chapter 3, the doctrine of informed consent dictates that patients are to be given complete, truthful information about all available treatments and courses of action concerning their health care. This information must be presented in a way that the patient can understand and must be given before any decisions are made or any procedures and treatments are instituted.

The principle of autonomy not only allows competent patients to choose a specific treatment but also grants patients the right to *refuse* treatment. The right to accept or refuse treatment is considered a component of the right to privacy implicit in the provisions of liberty of the United States Constitution.[4]

For patients who are incompetent, the rights granted through the principle of autonomy can be transferred to another individual through an advance directive, durable power of attorney, or living will. In these situations, any decisions made by the patient before the events that caused incompetence should be respected and implemented.

Examples of ethical conflicts involving the principle of autonomy include the following:

- The physician has a strong opinion concerning the appropriate course of treatment. The patient requests a different, nonconventional (but approved) therapy.
- A patient wants everything done. The family believes that treatment is futile and would prefer palliative care.
- The physician and the family believe that a patient is somewhat confused and no longer able to make wise decisions on his or her own. Psychological evaluation does not demonstrate incompetency.
- The patient elects to have no treatment and is aware that, as a result, he or she will die. The physician feels that he or she has a duty to continue to treat aggressively.
- The physician presents one treatment option to the patient, who agrees to the procedure. Some members of the nursing staff agree that this is an appropriate course of action, but are concerned because other possible options have not been presented or discussed.

Beneficence and Nonmaleficence

The principle of beneficence and nonmaleficence refers to the duty to promote and engage in activities that will have a positive effect on a patient while refraining from any activities that may cause harm. The earliest recognized framework on which this principle is based is the Hippocratic oath, in which a physician promises, in part, that he or she will use measures for the benefit of the sick according to his or her ability and judgment and will keep patients from harm and injustice.[5]

Although the intent of the principle of beneficence and nonmaleficence seems clear, in reality, the application of the principle can be challenging and can lead to ethical conflicts. The ethical question that is often raised is not whether a particular course of action is good or harmful but rather which course is better or *less* harmful than another. Examples of conflicts involving the principle of beneficence and nonmaleficence are as follows:

- A second course of chemotherapy is being considered for a young mother with cancer. The first course made her extremely ill, and she is terrified to go through it again. There is about a 50 percent chance that the cancer can be cured if the patient undergoes the chemotherapy.
- A patient has been severely burned. His hands and feet will probably need to be amputated. The patient, who has no family, is severely depressed and does not want to live. Through the use of aggressive therapy and medical care, physicians expect to be able to save his life.
- A patient has requested reconstructive surgery on her deformed legs and lower back because she believes she is ugly. According to one physician, the patient *might* be able to ambulate better after the surgery. Multiple operations would be needed, and there is a chance that the surgery would not be successful and that the patient might become a paraplegic.
- A patient with five small children has a family history of a serious disease. Both of her parents and three grandparents died of the disease. A new drug that has a 40 percent chance of preventing the disease has just been developed. The drug is very expensive and may have side effects. The patient has no medical insurance and would have to sell her home to obtain money to buy the drug.
- An elderly cancer patient has expressed many times that he has a fear of drugs and never wants to become addicted to narcotics. He is nearing death but may not die for several weeks. He is awake, alert, and constantly in a great deal of pain. Because of the patient's expressed fear of addiction and because he wants to be able to communicate, the physician has not increased the dosage of morphine. Family members are angry with the physician and believe that the patient should be relieved of his pain.

Justice

The final ethical principle is justice. This is the principle that is concerned with the distribution of services, care, and resources to those who are in need. It operates under the premise that people in similar circumstances should be treated similarly regardless of age, gender, race, creed, mental ability, social status, or financial resources.

The goal of this principle is to provide equitable treatment to everyone involved. However, health care resources *are* limited, and this goal is difficult to define and sometimes impossible to reach. As such, people involved in decision making must review information to determine the most just way to provide services, to ensure the greatest good to the people needing service.

Following are some examples of conflicts involving the principle of justice:

- A liver is available for transplantation. A possible recipient has had one transplant, which is failing rapidly. He continued to drink alcohol after the first transplant and has no plans to stop. He will die in a matter of days without the transplant. Another possible recipient is in no immediate danger of dying. He used to be a heavy drinker but stopped. He is active in Alcoholics Anonymous.
- A large sum of money has been donated for research on *one* disease. A university hospital must decide whether to use the money for research on a rare type of cancer that affects a few people in the community every year or to fund research on a common, mild problem that affects almost everyone in the community.
- A new "miracle" drug is being tested, and a community hospital has been asked to select one individual to enter a clinical trial for this drug. One proposed patient is 58 years old, single, wealthy, and a highly respected member of the community. Another possible patient, age 24, is the sole support of a spouse and three children, is known to gamble, and has a reputation for marital unfaithfulness.
- A baby was born with multiple, serious, life-threatening anomalies. His parents were advised not to seek aggressive treatment, but they located a university hospital that donated all treatments and services. The baby lived for 8 months and never left the neonatal intensive care unit. The total bill was $1.2 million. The mother is pregnant again. She has been told that this fetus has the same problems as her first baby. She has contacted the university hospital and is requesting that it accept this new baby for treatment when it is born.
- The father of Dr. E. is an industrialist who frequently makes donations to various hospitals. He recently gave a community hospital a large sum of money without restrictions as to how it was to be spent. Dr. E., a surgeon, wants to use the money to buy a piece of equipment, which only he and two other surgeons are likely to use. Dr. F. thinks that the money should be used to upgrade the hospital's children's immunization clinic, which is housed in a run-down storefront.

By specifically *naming* the conflict or ethical dilemma and by identifying which principle or principles may be involved, an institution can bring the issues of a case under discussion into clearer focus and therefore more easily address them.

Step 3: Clarify the Patient's Perspective

A clear understanding of the patient's perspective on the issues in question is essential to the process for ethical thinking and reflection. The wishes of the patient, if known, will play a central role in the case discussion and in the factors used to determine a recommended course of action.

The patient's desires can be determined through a number of sources. If the patient is competent, direct conversations will provide the desired information. If such a conversation has taken place, some questions that need to be asked are:

- Has the patient been fully informed about his or her medical condition?
- When did this conversation take place and who was involved?
- Have all the possible alternatives been presented and explained?
- Does the patient understand the consequences of each alternative?
- Has the patient had sufficient time to think about this information and reflect on all factors that might influence a decision?
- Has the patient made a clear statement about what he or she would want to happen in relation to treatment and care, and if so, what is the patient's desire?
- Has the patient's expressed desire remained the same over time?

If the patient is incompetent, information on the patient's desires can be obtained from a living will, if one is available, or through a person who has durable power of attorney for health care.

If neither of these options is available, it may be possible to obtain information concerning the patient's wishes from family members or friends, who may have knowledge of the patient's beliefs, religious convictions, and personal values. Although information from these sources may not be authorized through a legal directive, all pertinent information should at least be considered in an attempt to understand a patient's perspective on the situation being discussed.

Following are some questions that may help to clarify the patient's perspective:

- What is the patient's religious history?
- Does religion currently play an important role in the patient's life?
- Is there a particular religious point of view or directive in the patient's faith that addresses the present circumstance?
- Has a priest, minister, rabbi, or other religious leader been involved with the patient recently?

- Does information presented by an interested party conflict with the known religious or philosophical beliefs of the patient?
- What has the patient valued in his or her life?
- Which of the things that have been valued can be maintained and which would be lost through any particular course of action?
- What would the patient perceive as the economic, social, or psychological impacts of any decision?
- What has the patient stated in the past concerning terminal illness, life-sustaining measures, or so-called futile treatments?

The ultimate purpose in determination of the patient's wishes is to develop an understanding of the quality of life that the patient would find acceptable. *Quality of life* is a subjective term, and each individual not only has a different definition of the term but also different personal criteria for acceptability. For example, some patients may believe that there is no point in being "hooked up to machines" if there is no chance that they will regain mental function. Other patients may think that "where there is life, there is hope," and thus want everything possible done until death occurs. In another example, some patients may not wish to live if they become quadriplegic in a car accident. Others may believe that such an accident would be "God's will" and that there would be a divine purpose to the tragedy.

The determination of acceptable quality of life will assist those involved in the process for ethical thinking and reflection in developing a recommendation that considers the patient's preferences as well as the emotional and psychological factors that helped to establish those preferences.

Step 4: Identify the Treatment Alternatives

After all of the pertinent facts concerning the case have been gathered, the ethical concerns and conflicts stated, and the patient's perspectives identified, the next step in this process is to (1) list all of the possible alternatives for medical care and (2) identify the potential consequences of each.

General Categories of Treatments

Although the specifics concerning treatment alternatives vary depending on the individual case or category of cases being reviewed, there are four general categories into which the alternatives fall:

- Treat aggressively:
  - Initiate new therapies or modalities
  - Provide surgery
  - Use medications designed to cure
  - Use full CODE if patient goes into cardiopulmonary arrest

- Continue present level of treatment:
  - Maintain current level of medication
  - Maintain all presently used therapies and modalities
  - Maintain current CODE status
- Provide palliative care:
  - Use medications for pain control
  - Do not initiate therapy if condition deteriorates
  - Do not resuscitate (DNR) CODE status
- Withdraw from life-sustaining treatment:
  - Discontinue curative medications
  - Disconnect the ventilator
  - Discontinue artificial feeding and hydration
  - Do not resuscitate

Consequences of Treatments

The potential consequences of each of the treatment alternatives will also vary depending on the particular case. The action eventually taken will, however, ultimately have an effect on various groups and interested parties. In an evaluation of the potential consequences, it is helpful to ask some of the following questions (additional questions may be appropriate depending on the case):

- In relation to the patient:
  - What will be the emotional impact?
  - What will be the medical outcome of this treatment alternative?
  - Will the patient be cured?
  - Will the patient die immediately?
  - Will death be delayed because of this alternative?
  - Will the patient be relieved of pain and suffering?
  - How long might the patient live in this condition?
  - Is this alternative in keeping with the patient's wishes and values?
- In relation to the family, guardian, friends, or significant other:
  - What will be the emotional impact of this alternative?
  - What logistical problems may develop in relation to time and location of treatment, transportation, direct care, and so forth?
  - What financial impact will there be?
  - What is the comfort level with this alternative?
- In relation to the physicians and other health care workers:
  - How does this alternative compare with what is perceived as the medically indicated treatment?
  - What changes will there be in the type, level, and frequency of treatment modalities provided to the patient?
  - Will staffing levels need to be changed?

  - Will selection of this alternative create emotional difficulties for direct care providers?
- In relation to the institution and society:
  - What will be the financial impact of this alternative?
  - What is the length of time that the patient would likely remain at the facility?
  - Does the facility have the resources to provide the level of care required?
  - Are there any potential legal or liability issues?
  - In what ways might this treatment decision have an effect on general societal attitudes toward a particular health care procedure?
  - Will provision of this alternative for this patient affect the institution's ability to provide services for other patients?

Step 5: Determine What Is in the Best Interest of All Involved Parties

The determination of what is in the best interest of the parties involved is a challenge, because what is best for one individual is frequently not what is best for another. As a result, it is unlikely that one alternative will be ideal for all concerned or totally satisfactory to each member of a group. It is therefore important to try to understand the viewpoint of each person involved and to take this information into consideration in a discussion of the issues. The involved and concerned parties include:

- The patient
- The family, guardian, and friends
- The physician and other health care workers
- The health care organization and society

The following subsections discuss determining the best interests of each of these parties.

The Best Interest of the Patient

The most important determination in this step of the process is the determination of what is in the *patient's* best interest. This determination can be approached from two different perspectives, both of which are equally important.

First, what is in the best interest of the patient medically? This decision is based on a quantification of the benefits that can be achieved by applying medical knowledge and technical skills to the therapeutic needs and desires of the patient. It directly addresses the concepts of care versus cure, containment of disease, prevention or elimination of pain, relief of symptoms, and continuation of life. It answers the question, What appears to be *the* most appropriate course of medical care and treatment that can be provided?

The determination of what is in the patient's best interest medically must be based on sound reasoning, outcome probabilities, and clinical research statistics. It should not be based exclusively on a physician's personal judgment or on the perceptions of the medical staff concerning what would be an appropriate quality of life for the patient.

From the second perspective, what is the patient's concept of what is in his or her best interest? As discussed previously, the patient's desires, wishes, and values are an essential component of what the patient perceives as an appropriate level of care. Many of these factors are influenced by one's need for individual control, the need for the freedom to choose one's own destiny, and the desire to maintain personal dignity.

The patient is the *only* one who can truly know what types of care are tolerable and what quality of life is acceptable. Patients will consider the many pros and cons of the physical, emotional, and social context of the present or proposed medical experience and will weigh the potential benefits and burdens against their own needs and wants. Patients will also determine what is in their own best interest in relation to a personal concept of the meaning of life and from a framework of an individualized religious belief system.

A patient's determination of what is personally right may seem very wrong to other people. Acceptance of the patient's belief, in what is in his or her best interest, does not always imply agreement with that belief.

The Best Interest of the Family, Guardian, and Friends

The determination of what is in the best interest of family and friends may be the most challenging aspect of the fifth step in the process for ethical thinking and reflection. This is because of the various degrees of dependence and emotional closeness that these individuals will have with the patient. Although there may be next of kin whose interests must be considered paramount, there may also be others whose needs must be considered. In general, the actions that ultimately will be in the best interest of the individuals in this group are those that cause the least amount of emotional distress, the least social or logistical burden, the least guilt, and the least amount of conflict between members of the group.

The Best Interest of the Physician and Other Health Care Workers

The treatment alternative that will be in the best interest of the physician and other health care workers will be one that enables them to use their knowledge and skills to the best of their ability without compromising their integrity, principles, or moral beliefs. It will least disrupt their daily routine, have the least negative emotional consequences, and create the fewest differences of opinion among staff members.

The Best Interest of the Health Care Organization and Society

Identification of what is in the best interest of the health care organization and society not only involves looking at decisions in relation to any one patient but also involves examining the situation from a broader context. The treatment alternative that will be in the best interest of the institution will be one that can meet the medical needs of the patient, will have the least amount of financial impact and the least disruption of staffing, and will not have a deleterious effect on the ability to provide services to other individuals. In addition, it is important for the alternative to have minimal risk of litigation (for example, from an unhappy surviving family member who disagreed with a decision to allow a patient to die) and to have a limited risk of negative publicity (for example, avoiding expending large amounts of money to provide services to one patient while other people in the community need additional services).

For society, the determination of what is in the best interest is more vague and complex. In general, the best ethical alternative will be one from which the most people can ultimately gain (for example, by enhancing medical knowledge that can be used in other situations or by using limited resources to provide services to the greatest number of people).

Step 6: Select the Most Appropriate Alternative

The final step in the process of ethical thinking and reflection is to select *one* alternative or to suggest *one* course of action. The alternative selected should come closest to meeting the criteria for being in the best interest of the patient and should be the least problematic for all other involved individuals. This is the step in the process in which the most discussion and debate occur, when differences of opinion are voiced and conclusions are justified.

Selection of Alternatives in Case Consultations

In situations in which the process of selecting the most appropriate treatment is being used in case consultations, those involved in this process are asked to share their perceptions and to consider all information that has been presented so that they can make recommendations. The final committee recommendation is frequently reached through consensus, although a unanimous decision is not necessary.

It is important to note that a committee convened for the purpose of case consultation *does not* make decisions concerning patient treatment or care. Committees conduct case consultations for the purpose of guidance and counsel only and are responsible for helping patients, physicians, and others involved in the case to identify all the issues and to put some order into a difficult decision-making process. Case consultation is designed to provide an opportunity for a systematic analysis of what may be emotionally charged circumstances, not to provide definitive answers to difficult questions. The obligation to make an ultimate decision remains with the patient or with the responsible surrogate.

Selection of Alternatives in Educational Programs

When the process of ethical thinking and reflection is used during educational programs, this final step in the process—selecting alternatives in educational programs—is frequently the one that generates the most dialogue, the most involvement, and sometimes the most controversy. As participants become comfortable with the process and with taking part in biomedical ethics discussions, a wealth of diversified opinions and convictions may be cited.

Continued exposure to this process will help participants learn to discriminate between true ethical issues and problems that do not have an ethical component. It will help them to narrow the field of acceptable treatment alternatives and will enable them to identify which aspects of a situation have true relevance to any decisions that need to be made. As with case consultations, the final step in this process is to look at all the information that has been presented and to come to a conclusion as to which alternative for treatment appears to be best.

Summary

Ethical decisions, whether they are made by patients, family members, physicians, or other health care workers, are always made within the context of a personal value and belief system. There are many such systems among staff members in any institution and among the variety of patients who seek medical services. As such, there are a multitude of ways of looking at, and assessing ethical problems and a vast array of possible approaches to addressing ethical issues or making appropriate ethical choices. A formal, structured process for ethical thinking and reflection can assist in bringing together the common elements of these various ethical approaches so that individuals with different backgrounds can approach the task of ethical deliberation from a common framework.

The goals of a systematic process for ethical thinking and reflection are to provide a way for participants to identify all relevant factors related to a case or situation and to understand the various facts, conflicts, and alternatives that may have a significant impact on the provision of optimum patient care. This process enables participants to learn about the beliefs and philosophies of others without jeopardizing their own personal values or ethical beliefs.

References

1. Tillotson, F. Procedure for conducting case review by a medical/moral committee. Handout, Franciscan Health System Ethics Conference, Aston, PA, 1989.
2. Mappes, T. A., and Zembaty, J. S. *Biomedical Ethics*. 3rd ed. New York City: McGraw-Hill, 1991, p. 62.
3. Ross, J. W. *Handbook for Hospital Ethics Committees*. Chicago: American Hospital Publishing, 1986, pp. 26–27.
4. Annas, G. J., and Densberger, J. E. Competence to refuse medical treatment: autonomy vs. paternalism. *Toledo Law Review* 15(2):561, Winter 1984.
5. Mappes and Zembaty, p. 53.

Chapter Five

Biomedical Ethics Grand Rounds Programs

One educational format with which to expose interested individuals to the process of ethical thinking and reflection as well as to specific ethical issues and discussions is a biomedical ethics grand rounds program. A *biomedical ethics grand rounds program* is an event or series of events designed to educate physicians, nurses, and other health care workers on various aspects and ethical components of patient care, through both an observational and a participative format.

A biomedical ethics grand rounds program is a particularly useful tool for ethics education because it can be established in any size institution and because the format can be adapted to any size audience. Grand rounds can be implemented at any point along the continuum of a comprehensive biomedical ethics education plan, and it can be used to address any type of biomedical ethics issue or dilemma. In addition, the complexity and the content of a grand rounds program can be adapted to the learning needs of any target audience.

Simply put, a biomedical ethics grand rounds program is a forum in which ethical issues, dilemmas, and decisions concerning a particular patient or situation are presented and discussed. This chapter discusses in detail the following aspects of biomedical grand rounds:

- Program format
- Educational objectives and target audience
- Scheduling
- Coordinator's responsibilities
- Grand rounds pitfalls and what to do about them

An example of a grand rounds program is presented in the appendix at the end of this book.

Program Format

The specific program format of biomedical ethics grand rounds consists of five segments:

1. *Introduction and overview:* Either the coordinator of the program (usually the educator from the biomedical ethics committee) or the grand rounds panel moderator conducts the introduction and overview. A brief synopsis of the case is presented, the ethical issues to be addressed are identified, and the panel members are introduced.
2. *Presentations by panel members:* All panel members are asked to give a synopsis of the case from their own experience and in relation to their own particular disciplines.
3. *Issues clarification:* Once the case has been presented, the moderator then asks the audience to pose questions to the panel members. The questions will help to clarify the situation or help the audience to better understand the ethical dilemma concerning the case.
4. *Group discussion:* After all of the pertinent information has been presented and clarified, the moderator then leads an open-ended discussion concerning the conflicts, issues, problems, process, and outcomes of the case.
5. *Summary and conclusions:* During the final segment of grand rounds, the moderator summarizes the main points of the discussion, restates the ethical issues that were addressed, and formulates conclusions concerning the process of ethical thinking and reflection that took place in the context of the grand rounds program. (Note: It is not the responsibility of the moderator to draw conclusions about the outcome of the case. The conclusions that are drawn are specific to the content of the grand rounds program only.)

Because the time allotted for most grand rounds programs is limited, it is essential for the moderator to control each aspect of these five segments. (See figure 5-1.) For a one-hour grand rounds program it is recommended that the *introduction* take no more than five minutes. This should give the educator or moderator sufficient time to conduct the introductions of the panel members and to give the overview of the content, without taking too much time away from the rest of the program.

The *panel presentation* should take approximately 20 minutes, with half the time being allotted for the physician to present the medical facts and the rest of the time being divided among the other panel members (usually nursing and one or two other disciplines). It is important for the educator or moderator to tell the panel members, in advance, the amount of time allotted for each of their segments, so that they keep their presentations short and to the point.

Approximately 15 minutes should be allotted for *issues clarification* so that the audience has sufficient time to ask questions and to develop an understanding of the case or situation being presented. The final 20 minutes should be allotted for the *discussion* portion of the program. Often, the line between issues clarification and discussion is somewhat vague. It is appropriate for an audience member to ask for more clarification during the discussion portion and for the moderator to direct additional clarification questions to the appropriate panel member.

Figure 5-1. Recommended Time Allocations for Components of a One-Hour Grand Rounds Program

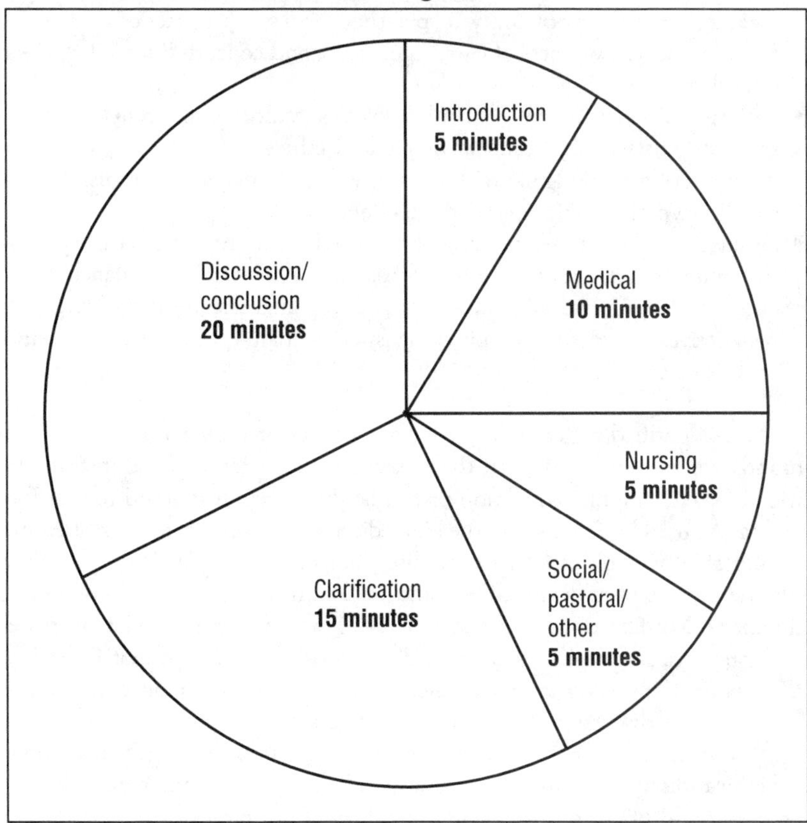

These time recommendations should be considered flexible and adaptable to the needs of the program and the audience. They may need to be adapted depending on the category of grand rounds being presented and should, obviously, be modified if the full amount of time for the program is longer or shorter than one hour.

Educational Objectives and Target Audience

Biomedical ethics grand rounds has certain specific educational objectives. These objectives include:

- Use of critical thinking skills
- Enhancement of the understanding of the ethical dimension of holistic patient care

- Provision of an overview of ethical theory and complex ethical issues
- Exposure of participants to a process used for ethical thinking and decision making, with an opportunity to put that process into practice
- Provision of an awareness of laws, regulations, and court decisions that affect ethical practice
- Exposure of participants to the philosophical, cultural, and religious diversity that exists in the realm of biomedical ethics
- Provision of a nonjudgmental format in which participants can discuss personal viewpoints, opinions, and experiences
- Facilitation of an understanding of the need for mutual respect of alternative points of view (This may help foster the skills needed to balance differences between personal ethical perspectives and the need to review *all* perspectives in order to provide compassionate, high-quality, ethically sound patient care.)

The identified target audience for any particular biomedical ethics grand rounds program will vary with the implementation status of the institution-wide biomedical ethics education plan. Initially, a modified grand rounds format can be used for members of the biomedical ethics committee so they become comfortable with retrospective case discussions and can practice before they use the process of ethical thinking and reflection in actual case consultation situations. Modifications might include using written cases rather than panel presentations, having less structured discussions, or—if the format is used as a component of the regularly scheduled biomedical ethics committee meeting—spreading the discussion over more than one session.

Once the biomedical ethics committee feels comfortable with this format for ethical discussions and wants to expand the program, grand rounds may be targeted to physicians and other members of the professional and clinical staff. These individuals will likely have a foundation for the medical and ethical issues being presented and may be familiar with specific information relevant to the case or topic being discussed.

In time, the goal should be to invite all members of the institutional staff to attend grand rounds programs. Although not all individuals who work in health care settings will have the opportunity to become directly involved in patient-related ethical issues, it is nevertheless useful and advantageous for everyone to have the opportunity to learn about ethical issues and to develop an understanding of the process used within the institution to address ethical problems.

As indicated in chapter 2, there are several reasons to include *all* levels of staff and individuals from every department in biomedical ethics education and specifically in grand rounds. First, as the concept of the health care team grows and evolves, it is essential for all members of that team to have an awareness of each of the components of service that combine to produce comprehensive, high-quality, compassionate care. As discussions of biomedical ethics and related topics have become more commonplace, it has become important to be certain that all members of the health care team have an awareness of biomedical ethics in general and of each institution's specific approach to ethical issues and problems.

A second reason to include all staff members is to provide a framework for action for staff members who become aware of problems or situations while on the job. Many nonclinical staff members interact with patients and family members on a daily basis. Any one of those individuals may encounter a situation with an ethical dimension. If all staff members are provided with the appropriate training to enable them to recognize these situations and know what to do about them, the likelihood of an ethical situation being unaddressed is diminished.

Finally, an understanding of biomedical ethics and ethical issues can be important for staff members in their personal lives. If a staff member or an employee's family member becomes a patient, any training in biomedical ethics in which employees have participated may help them to make knowledgeable and informed health care choices when the need arises.

In some cases, it may also be appropriate to invite members of the community or professionals from other facilities to attend these programs. Individuals such as staff members from local nursing homes, retirement communities, or home health agencies may benefit from exposure to the process used in ethical discussions that this format provides. Inclusion of these individuals will ultimately benefit any mutually shared patients and their families.

Scheduling

Various factors need to be taken into account when scheduling biomedical grand rounds. These include the frequency of the programs as well as their time and duration. The type of room in which the program will take place should also be considered.

Frequency

The number of times per year that a grand rounds program can be conducted will be influenced by several factors. The frequency of grand rounds may depend on the stage of development of the institutionwide biomedical ethics education program. Institutions with a well-developed ethics education program will probably be able to conduct the events more frequently than facilities whose programs are in the early stages.

The number of times per year that grand rounds can be conducted may also depend on the size of the institution. Larger facilities will likely encounter more cases that have an ethical dilemma and will therefore have a greater pool of cases and situations for presentation.

Frequency of grand rounds also will depend on the number and types of other biomedical ethics in-service programs being conducted as well as on the amount of time that staff has available to coordinate the program. An additional factor may be the availability and willingness of staff to participate on a panel.

Each institution should establish a set frequency for grand rounds that meets its own needs and requirements. Programs conducted semiannually, quarterly, or monthly can be equally effective and educationally sound.

Duration and Time

A one-hour program is recommended for grand rounds. Any less time does not allow for adequate presentation or discussion, and any more time presents difficulties for staff to attend because of work obligations.

Although grand rounds can be conducted at any point during the day, holding the program over the lunch hour seems to work well. (A free lunch to attendees would, of course, draw a crowd, but an invitation to staff to brown-bag, with complimentary beverages and dessert, is also a nice touch.)

Room Design

Another consideration in scheduling is selecting a room that can be arranged to provide maximum audience interaction. Although a theater-style seating arrangement can be used for grand rounds and is conducive to accommodating the largest number of people in a given space, this arrangement tends to thwart effective audience interactions. An arrangement with tables and chairs that are angled toward the center of the room is more appropriate for group discussion, which is a key component of grand rounds. (See figure 5-2.)

Coordinator's Responsibilities

To be certain that all the necessary components for a grand rounds program have been addressed, it is recommended that one individual from the biomedical ethics committee (ideally an educator) be assigned the role of grand rounds program coordinator. A program design format similar to the one illustrated in figure 5-3 should be developed and used to ensure that all the details of the program are addressed.

The grand rounds event coordinator has several specific responsibilities. They are:

- Selecting the category of presentation
- Selecting the specific topic or case for presentation
- Selecting and preparing members of the grand rounds panel
- Preparing publicity and audience materials

Figure 5-2. Ideal Seating Arrangement for Grand Rounds

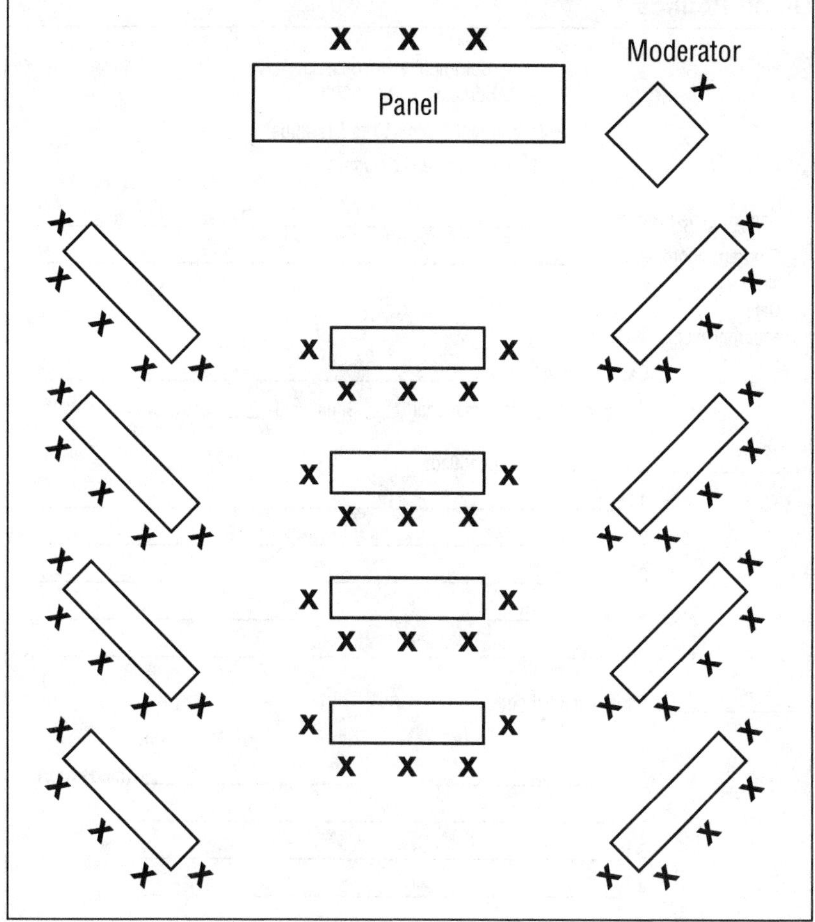

- Handling the logistical details
- Evaluating and summarizing the program

These responsibilities are explained in greater detail in the following subsections.

Selecting the Category of Presentation

There are three basic categories for biomedical ethics grand rounds presentations: informational, situational, and retrospective case review. A thorough, ongoing biomedical ethics education plan should use a combination of all three of these categories to provide the audience with a global and comprehensive overview of biomedical ethics topics and issues.

Figure 5-3. Sample Program Design Form for Biomedical Ethics Grand Rounds

Community Hospital
Hometown, PA 19000

Biomedical Ethics Grand Rounds

Program Design

Date of scheduled event: ______________________ Time: _____ to _____

Program coordinator: ______________________________________

Date accomplished: Task:

__________ Case/topic selected: ______________________________

Category: ___ Informational ___ Situational ___ Case Review

__________ Objectives/issues identified:

1. ______________________________
2. ______________________________
3. ______________________________
4. ______________________________
5. ______________________________

__________ Panel established:

Name Title Phone No.

1. ______________________________ (moderator)
2. ______________________________
3. ______________________________
4. ______________________________
5. ______________________________

__________ Pre-grand rounds panel meeting scheduled: ______________

__________ Room reserved

__________ Food ordered

__________ Audiovisual equipment scheduled

__________ Notices prepared/distributed

__________ Handouts prepared/duplicated

__________ Evaluations prepared/duplicated

__________ CME/CEU credits arranged

__________ Other: ______________________________
____

Informational Presentations

Informational grand rounds programs provide the audience with information that they will need to understand the basic components of ethical theory and process. They cover content areas and focus on facts rather than on interpretation.

Following are some sample titles of informational grand rounds programs:

- *An Overview of Biomedical Ethics History:* This program or programs would cover information concerning the development of the biomedical ethics movement as well as the role of the patient in health care decision making. An overview would present information on the documentation of patient choice through consent forms, durable power of attorney, or living wills. It would also include information on right-to-die issues, life-sustaining treatments, and medical futility. (This historical topic could easily be divided into several grand rounds events.)
- *What Is a Biomedical Ethics Committee and How Does It Function?* This program would cover the roles and responsibilities of the biomedical ethics committee as well as the committee membership and the process for accessing the committee. It might also include any information relevant to the institution's process of arranging for ethics committee consults.
- *The Process for Addressing an Ethical Dilemma:* This program would provide information to the participants about the steps and procedure for reviewing ethical situations and cases (See chapter 4.)
- *The Language and Terminology of Biomedical Ethics:* This presentation would cover words and phrases that are common to the discussion of biomedical ethics topics. (See the glossary at the end of this book.)
- *Policies that Address Ethical Issues:* In this program, existing institutional policies that have an ethical dimension would be reviewed and discussed.
- *Laws and Regulations: How Do They Affect Biomedical Ethics?* This program would cover topics such as required request (regulations requiring discussion of organ transplant in appropriate situations), informed consent, and the Patient Self-Determination Act, as well as any applicable state laws or local regulations.
- *Court Cases and Their Impact on Biomedical Ethics Practice:* This program would cover specific cases that have resulted either in enhanced awareness of biomedical ethics issues or in precedents being set concerning the handling of certain types of situations.

It is practical to use informational presentations for programs conducted in the early phases of any grand rounds educational effort. These programs can provide the foundation and framework for discussions of specific issues and applied ethics that will occur in future programs. (See the bibliography and resources at the end of the book for information concerning topics for informational grand rounds presentations.)

Situational Presentations

Situational grand rounds presentations address either a particular ethical problem or a series of related topics. They include presentation of various examples or cases pertaining to that problem or topic and a discussion of their impact on patients, family members, and the health care team.

Some examples of titles for situational presentations are:

- *Ethical Issues Related to Organ and Tissue Donation:* This presentation would cover topics such as the criteria for brain death, the Anatomical Gift Act, and the process to be used when approaching the family of a deceased individual to discuss organ and tissue donation.
- *The Noncompliant Patient:* In this presentation, examples of noncompliant patients would be discussed along with the difficulties that these patients present for the staff. (See the appendix.)
- *Euthanasia and Assisted Suicide:* This program would cover the difference between active euthanasia (an act that causes death) and passive euthanasia (not doing something, which allows a death to occur) and would give examples of each. It would also cover different views on whether physicians should assist terminal and chronically ill patients to take their own lives.
- *Treatment of the Very Low Birth Weight Infant:* This program would cover the pros and cons of providing intensive care to extremely small infants as well as the ethical issues that arise in making these treatment choices.

Situational grand rounds programs enable participants to be exposed to an overview of various points of view related to a wide range of subjects. They are particularly useful if the members of the target audience are individuals who are in the early stages of their biomedical ethics education.

Situational presentations also offer an opportunity to respond to issues that are hot topics in the news. (See the bibliography and resources at the end of this book for information concerning topics for situational grand rounds presentations.)

Retrospective Presentations

Undoubtedly, the most common and probably the most useful type of biomedical ethics grand rounds program category is that of the retrospective case review. In this type of program, the information that is presented and discussed pertains to the ethical issues surrounding the case of one particular patient. Initially, the case that is presented can be hypothetical (see chapter 8) or one taken from the literature. Later, when there is an increased comfort level with the types of discussions that take place during retrospective case reviews, the case can be about someone who has actually been a patient in the facility in which the grand rounds program is being held.

The discussion in retrospective case reviews centers on actual ethical issues experienced by the patient, the family, and the medical community. Although confidentiality must be maintained throughout, this type of discussion covers the dilemmas that arose and the way that the situation was ultimately handled and resolved. In many cases, some of the members of the audience for a retrospective case review will be individuals who were directly involved with the case. They will have experienced firsthand the conflicts that arose, the emotions that were generated, and the results of decisions that were made. Thus, a retrospective case review format provides the opportunity for individuals to share their experiences with other staff members and to voice their professional and emotional reactions to the events that occurred.

Some examples of titles of retrospective case reviews are:

- *The Case of Mr. A. An Alert, Oriented Patient Who Requested to Be Removed from the Respirator . . . against Family Wishes*
- *The Case of Mr. B. A Terminally Ill Cancer Patient Who Wanted Everything Done and Every Possible Treatment Known to Medical Science*
- *The Case of Baby C. An Infant Who Was Nonresponsive at Birth and Suffered Severe Brain Damage after Being Resuscitated*

Retrospective case review grand rounds programs are beneficial not only for staff members who provide direct patient care but also for other staff members, in that they can help to provide an understanding of how ethical theory and content can be applied in actual settings.

Selecting the Specific Topic or Case for Presentation

As previously stated, the selection of a topic or case for grand rounds is the responsibility of the grand rounds program coordinator (with input and assistance from the biomedical ethics committee or a subgroup of that committee). Topics should be varied, timely, and of interest and significance to the staff who will be invited to attend the programs. One method of obtaining ideas for grand rounds programs is to solicit input directly from the staff concerning their needs and interests. (See figure 5-4.)

A second method is to review the records of any actual case consultations that the biomedical ethics committee has conducted since the previous grand rounds event. This will provide information about specific cases that may be appropriate to review and about the types of issues that recently have had a significant impact on the institution.

Selecting and Preparing Panel Members

Proper selection and preparation of panel members are essential to a successful grand rounds presentation. Panel members must know the topic or case well enough to be able to speak about it from their own experience, and they must also be able to spontaneously answer questions from the audience.

Figure 5-4. Sample Request Form for Suggestions from Staff for Grand Rounds Programs

Community Hospital
Hometown, PA 19000

Memo: (Date) ____________________

To: (Appropriate staff) ____________________

From: (Program coordinator) ____________________

Re: Suggestions for the next Biomedical Ethics Grand Rounds

The next grand rounds program is scheduled for (date).
As always, we feel that it is important to present cases and issues that are important to our staff and to Community Hospital in general. As such, you are invited to submit a suggestion for a topic or case that you believe would be of interest.

Please return the following form to me by (date).

- -

Your name (optional)

Phone no. (optional)

Case/issue that you would like to see presented at grand rounds:

____

____

____

Reason that you feel that this would be appropriate to present:

____

____

____

Would you be willing to be a grand rounds panel member?

____ Yes ____ No

For a one-hour grand rounds program, the panel should consist of no more than three or four members. The specific type of individuals who are best suited to be on the panel will depend largely on the type and category of the presentation being held. For retrospective case reviews, the panel generally should include the primary physician and someone from the nursing staff. Other members may include a consulting physician, a risk manager, a social worker, a chaplain, someone from one of the therapies (physical, respiratory, occupational, for example), or any other individual who had direct involvement with the patient and who was aware of the ethical dimensions of the case.

Besides the panel members themselves, there needs to be an individual who will moderate the grand rounds program. This individual may be an educator, a physician, an administrator, or someone from the biomedical ethics committee.

The moderator may also be a trained ethicist (either an in-house expert or someone brought in from the outside). The advantages of using a trained ethicist are that such an individual is an expert in the theory and philosophy of ethical issues and would have a knowledge base that probably would be much more extensive than that of members of the regular institutional staff. An ethicist should be very comfortable with the language and terminology of ethical issues and would consequently be able to guide the learning and discussions in a systematic manner. Finally, a trained ethicist should be able to maintain a level of objectivity, an essential ingredient for discussions that may have a high degree of emotion.

Some disadvantages of using an ethicist are the risks that the individual may be too philosophical, may be perceived to be overly theoretical, or may be out of touch with applied ethics. Ethicists brought in from outside the institution would not have the advantage of knowing the culture of the facility, which may negatively affect their ability to relate appropriately to the panel or the audience.

In addition, ethicists who have received extensive training in the field will—consciously or unconsciously—bring to any discussion their own personal biases, educational backgrounds, and points of view. If an ethicist is to be used as grand rounds moderator, care should be taken to select someone who will appreciate all ethical perspectives.

It is wise for the program coordinator to meet with the moderator and the entire panel before the grand rounds to establish the moderator's role, review the content of each member's presentation, discuss the ethical issues that will be addressed, and confirm the time constraints under which the program will operate.

Preparing Publicity and Audience Materials

Well-designed publicity and audience handout materials are important components for successful grand rounds programs. They provide the motivation for people to attend the event and the supporting information that will assist participants to understand the material being presented during the event.

Announcements and Notices

Appropriate publicity in the form of announcements or notices is essential to ensure that staff members are invited to the grand rounds program and that they receive sufficient information to understand the scope of the program content and its objectives. Notices should include all logistical details, including date, time, location, and, if necessary, registration requirements. A brief description of the type of program—instructional, situational, or case review—and basic information concerning the ethical issues to be addressed are also appropriate.

Care needs to be taken to ensure that the information contained in any announcements or notices does not inadvertently breach confidentiality. It is wise for the program coordinator to have the content of any announcements and notices reviewed by the biomedical ethics committee, the institution's risk manager or attorney, or the medical director before distribution to be certain that the content and subject matter is appropriately phrased. Sample announcements are provided in figures 5-5, 5-6, and 5-7 (pp. 91–93).

Handouts

Because a grand rounds program is intended to cover a significant amount of information or ethical content in a relatively short time, it is often useful to provide members of the audience with a handout, which gives them the highlights of the subject or case, an overview of the ethical issues to be discussed, and any other additional information that will enable them to understand and participate in the process. See figures 5-8, 5-9, and 5-10 (pp. 94–96).

Such a handout might include the following:

- A list of the panel members and an identification of their role in relation to the case
- A summary of the medical history of the patient or patients
- A synopsis of the family dynamics
- An overview of available treatment options
- An outline of the main points or issues that the panel will discuss

The handout might also include definitions of some of the key ethical terms and phrases likely to be used in the course of the impending discussion. Providing audience members with this type of handout helps to keep the program focused and assists in guiding the audience toward constructive group participation.

Figure 5-5. Sample Grand Rounds Announcement: Informational Presentation

Community Hospital
Hometown, PA 19000

Biomedical Ethics Grand Rounds

Panel Presentation

Tuesday
March 6
12:00 to 1:00 p.m.

Conference Room A

The panel will present information concerning:

1. The role, composition, and function of Community Hospital's biomedical ethics committee

2. A standardized process for ethical thinking, reflection, and case review

3. The procedure used for addressing specific ethical issues for Community Hospital patients

Attendees will have an opportunity to ask questions and share personal views and perspectives

Please feel free to brown-bag your lunch
Beverages and dessert will be provided

Figure 5-6. Sample Grand Rounds Announcement: Situational Presentation

Community Hospital
Hometown, PA 19000

Biomedical Ethics Grand Rounds

The Noncompliant Patient

Friday
July 12
12:00 to 1:00 p.m.

Conference Room B

The panel will consist of representatives from:

Home Health
Rehabilitation Services
Hemodialysis

Please join us as we discuss:

1. Examples of noncompliant patients
2. Our ethical and legal obligations to these individuals
3. Safety issues
4. The frustrations encountered by staff in their efforts to provide service

This program is open to all interested Community Hospital staff

Please feel free to bring your lunch;
we will supply soda and cookies

*Physicians: As an organization accredited by ACCME,
ABC University School of Medicine certifies
that this educational program meets the criteria for one hour in Category I,
provided it is completed as designed.*

Figure 5-7. Sample Grand Rounds Announcement: Retrospective Case Review

Community Hospital
Hometown, PA 19000

Biomedical Ethics Grand Rounds

Friday
October 19
12:00 to 1:00 p.m.

Conference Room A

Retrospective Case Review
and
Panel Discussion

Please join us as our panel presents the case of an alert, oriented, competent patient who wanted to be removed from a respirator against the strong wishes of his family.

The panel members include his primary physician, a social worker, and a member of the nursing staff who was involved in his direct care.

This program is open to all Community Hospital Staff

Luncheon will be provided

Seating is limited.
Please call ext. 1234 to register

Figure 5-8. Sample Grand Rounds Handout: Informational Presentation

Community Hospital
Hometown, PA 19000

Biomedical Ethics Grand Rounds

March 6
12:00 to 1:00 p.m.

Biomedical Ethics at Community Hospital: An Overview

Panel:

Mr. John Jones
President/CEO, Community Hospital
Chair of the Biomedical Ethics Committee

Ms. Mert Miller, R.N., J.D.
Director of Risk Management

Miss Louisa Lengrini, M.S.W.
Director of Social Services

Mr. Robert Reed, M.D., Ph.D.
Professor of Ethics
Hometown University
(Moderator)

Our grand rounds program today is designed to provide you with an overview of Community Hospital's approach to biomedical ethics as well as ethical issues you may encounter on the job.

The discussion will cover the structure, role, and function of the biomedical ethics committee as well as information concerning how you and your patients can get help from the committee if needed.

In addition, we will introduce you to a process that is used by the committee to organize thinking on the various components of ethical issues. We encourage you to use this process as you reflect on issues that you may encounter.

Please feel free to ask the panel members for clarification of any point or to answer specific questions concerning ethical decision making.

Figure 5-9. Sample Grand Rounds Handout: Situational Presentation

Community Hospital
Hometown, PA 19000

Biomedical Ethics Grand Rounds

July 12
12:00 to 1:00 p.m.

The Noncompliant Patient

Our ethics grand rounds discussion today centers on the issue of noncompliant patients—those individuals who complicate their care by not following instructions, not getting treatments that they need, leaving the hospital against medical advice, or choosing to live in "unsafe" or "unhealthy" environments, which compromise them medically.

Case examples:

Mrs. L. is a patient who has multiple sclerosis. She has been admitted to our hospital nine times over the past year and a half. The patient chooses to live alone with minimal support. Staff, however, believe that her inability to adequately provide self-care results in her multiple hospitalizations. A psychological evaluation showed that she is competent.

Mr. B. had a stroke and was subsequently admitted to our rehabilitation unit. He needed extensive treatment and therapy. The patient was uncooperative in all aspects of his care and left the hospital against medical advice. He was later readmitted following an amputation of his leg. The amputation had to be done as a result of improper self-care.

Mr. T. is a diabetic who receives hemodialysis treatments. He often does not arrive at scheduled times, and staff have asked the police to check on him on numerous occasions.

Questions:

1. What is our ethical and moral obligation to these patients?
2. What is the impact of these individuals on our staff?
3. What is the impact of these patients on health care resources?

Please feel free to ask questions and join in the discussion.

Reminder: All information being discussed during grand rounds must remain confidential. Thank you.

Figure 5-10. Sample Grand Rounds Handout: Retrospective Case Review

Community Hospital
Hometown, PA 19000

Biomedical Ethics Grand Rounds

October 19
12:00 to 1:00 p.m.

The Case of Mr. Z.

Mr. Z. was a 75-year-old man who was admitted to Community Hospital for a routine chemotherapy treatment. During the treatment, he experienced respiratory distress and was placed on a mechanical respirator from which he subsequently could not be weaned.

The patient was happily married. He had two grown, involved children.

Mr. Z. was awake, alert, and oriented. He requested several times to be removed from the respirator, and on more than one occasion he attempted to remove the tube on his own. The patient was fully aware that removal of the mechanical support would result in his death.

His family did not want the respirator removed. His wife claimed that he was confused.

Mr. Z. did not have a living will or any other form of advance directive.

The health care professionals involved in the case felt very confused and conflicted, as if they were caught in the middle. They wanted to comply with the patient's wishes but recognized that the lack of agreement from the family members was an issue of concern.

This case is also unusual in that most termination of respirator cases involve patients who are either brain dead or in a coma. Mr. Z., on the other hand, was not only conscious but also aware of and involved in the decision-making process.

Handling Logistical Details

Another consideration for the program coordinator in planning a grand rounds program is assumption of responsibility for the logistical details of the event. To be as certain as possible that the grand rounds program runs smoothly, it is important for the program coordinator to handle the logistical details. For example, the coordinator should expect to be responsible for:

- Scheduling the room
- Communicating the desired furniture arrangement
- Ordering the food
- Ordering any microphones or audiovisual equipment necessary
- Obtaining continuing education unit (CEU)/continuing medical education (CME) credits
- Duplicating materials

Evaluating and Summarizing the Program

Finally, it is also the obligation of the program coordinator to evaluate and summarize the event. The evaluation should have two components.

1. *Audience evaluation:* Each member of the audience should be asked to complete an event evaluation. This will provide information about individual perspectives concerning the learning experience, which will then be useful in adapting and planning future programs to meet these identified needs. (See figure 5-11.)
2. *Coordinator review:* The program coordinator should summarize his or her observations about the grand rounds, including all pertinent content issues and any comments or suggestions from the moderator or panel members. (See figure 5-12.)

Information concerning both of these evaluations should then be provided to the members of the biomedical ethics committee. This will enable them to be kept aware of the issues presented, the content reviewed, and any additional identified learning needs of the staff. The evaluations can also serve as a guide in the planning of other components of the comprehensive biomedical ethics education program.

Pitfalls of Grand Rounds and What to Do about Them

As is the case in any other educational program, there may be moments in grand rounds when things do not go smoothly or as anticipated. It is therefore

Figure 5-11. Sample Biomedical Ethics Grand Rounds Evaluation Form

Community Hospital
Hometown, PA 19000

Biomedical Ethics Grand Rounds

Evaluation

Name of attendee (optional): ______________________________

Date of program: ______________________________

Please rate this grand rounds program on the following questions:
(5 = to the highest degree; 1 = not at all)

1. How well did the program meet the stated objectives? 5 4 3 2 1
2. Did you learn new information? 5 4 3 2 1
3. Will the information be useful to you in your job? 5 4 3 2 1
4. Was the program interesting? 5 4 3 2 1
5. Was the handout helpful? 5 4 3 2 1
6. Was the information presented in a clear and concise manner? 5 4 3 2 1

Comments/concerns/questions: ______________________________

____

____

Suggestions for future grand rounds programs: ______________________________

____

____

Figure 5-12. Sample Biomedical Ethics Grand Rounds Program Coordinator Review

Community Hospital
Hometown, PA 19000

Biomedical Ethics Grand Rounds

Program Coordinator Review

Date of program: ______________

Total number of attendees: _____

Number of physicians who attended: _____

Summary of panel presentations:

Main points and ethical issues discussed:

Key areas and questions raised by the audience:

Conclusions:

Recommendations for content or format of future programs:

Report prepared by: ______________________________

Date: ______________

wise to have an understanding of the common types of potential problems and an idea of how to address them. Some potential problems are:

- Not enough participation
- Too much participation
- Confidentiality lapses
- High levels of emotions
- Insufficient time
- Participant confusion

Not Enough Participation

Situations where no one talks are a relatively common problem in the early phases of the implementation of grand rounds as a component of any biomedical ethics education program. The idea of participating in complex ethical discussions in a heterogeneous group setting can be intimidating at first. Participants need to be reassured of the following:

- Everyone's opinion is respected and has value.
- There are no wrong questions or inappropriate answers.
- Differences of opinion concerning ethical problems as well as differences in beliefs concerning how situations should be handled are expected and encouraged.
- Deeper personal and group understanding of ethical issues will come from the sharing of thoughts, feelings, and ideas.

Before the beginning of any grand rounds event, it is wise for the program coordinator to prepare a set of open-ended questions that can be used by the moderator to stimulate audience participation. It may also be helpful for the coordinator to ask members of the biomedical ethics committee, who presumably have had prior experience in ethical discussions, to attend grand rounds programs and be contributing members of the audience.

Too Much Participation

After staff members have attended one or more grand rounds programs and develop a comfort level with the process and the content, there is a risk that more people will want to participate in the discussion than time will allow. Audience participation can become very involved, with many individuals wanting to state an opinion or ask a question. In some cases, the panel or the moderator may be overshadowed if "point–counterpoint" discussions begin to occur between members of the audience. Although it is clearly the intention of grand rounds to include as many people as possible in the discussion, it is the obligation—and challenge—of the moderator to maintain some semblance of control, to keep participants on track, and to diffuse any potential conflicts that may arise as differences of opinion are voiced.

Confidentiality Lapses

As mentioned earlier, it is important to keep confidentiality in mind in relation to all aspects of grand rounds programs. It is recommended that all patients be referred to by some sort of code, such as Mr. X. or Ms. Z. However, even when this is done, frequently there is sufficient information presented in the discussion for attendees at a grand rounds to figure out who the patient really is.

Frequently, there are people in the audience who attend the program because they are aware that a particular patient is being discussed. Sometimes, in an effort to make a specific point about this patient (especially if there is an issue about which they have strong feelings), they may inadvertently use the patient's name. It is also possible that a member of the panel could make this same mistake. It is therefore wise to include a reminder about the need for confidentiality in any introduction to the grand rounds presentation and to write such a reminder on the handout.

High Levels of Emotion

The subject matter and the varied opinions that are explored can create intense emotional responses from both the panel members and the audience during grand rounds. In some cases, these emotions may be the result of unresolved issues related to the specific case being presented, or they may also reflect personal issues related to similar situations that the individual has experienced in the past.

These emotions can range from frustration, sadness, or anger to extreme joy or a high level of satisfaction for a job well done. Different individuals may have opposite emotional reactions to the same piece of information. As a result, there may be many emotional experiences and expressions happening simultaneously.

Although emotional responses per se should not be entirely discouraged during grand rounds, it is important to remember that the program is part of an educational group process, which is not intended to be a type of group therapy. Consequently, the moderator for the program must always be aware of the emotional climate and must be prepared to address and, if necessary, diffuse any potential problems that may be developing. It may also be helpful to have a plan (such as assistance from the social services or pastoral care staff) to address the follow-up needs of any participants who wish to continue to process their emotions once the grand rounds event has concluded.

Insufficient Time

Although a one-hour program usually meets the scheduling needs of both the panel members and the staff who will attend grand rounds, it often proves to be a small amount of time in which to cover all that needs to be included to make the event truly meaningful. Often, the time allotted for the program is over just as the discussion really gets going. However, it is usually not practical to allow additional time during the event. Some suggestions for continuing the flow of interactions after the grand rounds include:

- Encouraging supervisors to include a follow-up discussion concerning grand rounds in their regularly scheduled department meetings
- Establishing small discussion groups for the purpose of continued dialogue and reflection
- Encouraging informal discussions among interested staff

In addition, some of the issues that have been raised or content areas needing additional clarification can become topics for subsequent biomedical ethics education in-service programs or future grand rounds programs.

Participant Confusion

Although participants who leave the grand rounds program with more questions than answers may appear to be a problem, in reality, their questions can be a positive outcome of this educational effort. One of the main purposes of grand rounds is to stimulate ethical thinking and awareness. If participants leave the program with questions and the need to learn more about ethics in general or about the application of biomedical ethics in particular, then the grand rounds has accomplished an important goal.

It is important to reassure participants, however, that leaving the program with some unresolved feelings and unanswered questions is expected and that grand rounds is a tool to stimulate thinking, not a process designed to draw definitive conclusions concerning ethical issues. It may be helpful to provide participants with a list of resources or information concerning how they can obtain additional information about the topics presented during the grand rounds program.

Summary

Grand rounds can be an efficient, effective, meaningful method of providing health care workers with information on both theory and application strategies concerning biomedical ethics. The format of grand rounds provides opportunities for participants not only to learn about specific cases and situations that have had an impact on their own facility, but also to become familiar with laws, regulations, medical advancements, and societal developments that have had a broader impact on the ethical decision-making components of health care.

Biomedical ethics grand rounds is intended to be both interdisciplinary and interactive. This allows participants to use communication skills, practice a process for ethical thinking and reflection, and be exposed to the various ethical viewpoints and philosophies that make up an institutional ethical matrix. It is important to remember that the intention of grand rounds is to raise the ethical awareness of the participants, not to provide them with answers to complex ethical questions.

Chapter Six

Educational Tools

Until recent years, biomedical ethics, death and dying, and terminal illness were not, as a general rule, openly discussed, nor were educational programs conducted to specifically address these topics and the complex issues that they generate. Now, however, these and other related topics are routinely covered in the mass media as well as in lectures, group discussions, and educational courses.

As awareness of these issues has increased, so too has the need for educational tools that can be used to enable interested participants not only to expand their knowledge but also to learn how to integrate theoretical and cognitive understanding with affective and applied skills. As an educational tool, a comprehensive biomedical ethics education program needs to include a wide variety of events and activities; these should be specifically designed to enable individuals to explore the various elements that shape their perception of ethical issues.

Such educational experiences can range from short, nonthreatening events to longer, complex, and emotionally challenging activities. They may involve topics such as communication, end-of-life decisions, ethical awareness, and values clarification, or any combination thereof. These experiences should be designed to foster interaction among the participants, stimulate thinking, encourage personal awareness and assessment, and challenge participants to be open to different and varied ethical perspectives.

Chapters 6, 7, and 8 of this book provide educational tools that can be used to conduct these types of activities. It is not intended that *all* of these tools should be incorporated into a biomedical ethics education program. The educator or the other individuals who establish such a program should select those activities that would be appropriate to meet their learning objectives or the needs of the target audience.

In addition to the specific educational tools provided, the chapters also contain information on how to use the tools as well as copies of any handouts that may be needed. (Note: Tools and handouts may be copied for use in educational programs.)

The Nature of Structured Learning Activities

Structured learning activities are planned and organized educational experiences designed to teach or reinforce a particular concept or skill. They are conducted with specific learning goals in mind and offer participants an opportunity to become actively involved in a process that will enhance their knowledge base and their ability to apply that knowledge.

In biomedical ethics education, structured learning activities are useful in that they also enable participants to examine feelings about ethical issues, develop an awareness of different approaches to ethical dilemmas, and explore how different ethical situations might be handled, without leaving the safety of an educational environment.

Format

Each of the structured learning activities offered at the end of this chapter is presented in the following format. This format is offered as a guide, with the recommendation that the facilitator adapt and personalize the activity to meet the needs of individual groups. (Note: In this context, the word *facilitator* is used to designate the individual who is actually conducting the event. This may or may not be the educator, the person usually responsible for establishing and coordinating the *entire* biomedical ethics education program.)

- *Title:* The name of the activity (which in most cases gives an indication of the content area to be addressed)
- *Goals:* A summary of the broad learning objectives of the activity
- *Category:* An indication of one or more topic areas—in addition to "general awareness of ethical issues"—for which this activity would be a suitable form of reinforcement; suggests which activities are suitable to reinforce a particular learning need
- *Group size:* The recommended group size for maximum learning effectiveness
- *Minimum time:* The least amount of time needed to adequately conduct all components of the activity
- *Supplies:* Any handouts, materials, equipment, or room specifications needed
- *Procedure:* Step-by-step guidelines on how to conduct the activity
- *Discussion:* Questions the facilitator can use at the conclusion of the activity to promote a discussion about the learning that took place and the participants' reactions to the experience

The Facilitator's Role

The facilitator's role is divided into three parts: before the activity, during the activity, and after the activity.

Before the Activity

Before the activity starts, the facilitator is responsible for reviewing the structured learning activity and for determining whether there needs to be any modifications to the activity for the type of group that will be involved. In some cases, the facilitator is also responsible for the initial selection of the activity to be done. In these cases, the facilitator needs to assess the learning needs of the particular group and then review reasons why an activity would be helpful, in order to select an activity that is compatible with those factors.

A second and extremely important task of the facilitator before the start of an activity is advance preparation—familiarization with the activity to be conducted. The facilitator must review the goals, procedures, and discussion questions. For facilitators who may not have extensive backgrounds in a particular topic area, preactivity research and readings may be appropriate. (See the bibliography and resources at the end of the book for information that may help meet this requirement.)

Advance preparation also may require the gathering of supplies and materials that will be used in the activity.

During the Activity

The first thing that the facilitator does during the activity is to prepare the learning group to work together in the activity. Groups that have not previously been together should be encouraged to have the group members conduct self-introductions or participate in a brief activity that serves as an ice breaker before they are introduced to the activity. Groups whose members know each other can begin with an introduction to the activity itself (including a review of content area if necessary).

At this time, it is important for the facilitator to inform the participants that their level of participation and disclosure in any aspect of the activity is a matter of personal choice. Participation and involvement should be voluntary, and people should not be forced to do anything that makes them uncomfortable or that they find disturbing.

In addition, participants also must be made aware that a structured learning activity is *not* a therapy session. Although there may indeed be a therapeutic benefit to the experience, the activity itself is intended to be of educational benefit only.

The facilitator then conducts the activity, being careful to follow the procedure and to maintain the time schedule. Although many of the activities presented at the end of this chapter can be adapted to flexible time frames, it is up to the facilitator to be certain, no matter how long the total event takes, that there is adequate time at the end for discussion and summary.

The discussion portion of a structured learning activity is an important component of the learning process. It enables the participants to express their individual responses and feelings about the experience while providing a forum for those individuals to compare and contrast the general learning that has taken place. During the discussion, it is important that the facilitator validate the thoughts and feelings of everyone by stressing that there are no wrong feelings or inappropriate reactions. Participants need to know that even though everyone will not have the same reaction to the activity, each reaction and response is valid and respected.

The final responsibility of the facilitator during the activity is to summarize what actually happened and what the participants' responses were to the activity, and to compare both to the learning goals outlined before the activity. A formal program evaluation also may be conducted at this time.

After the Activity

After the structured learning activity, it is the responsibility of the facilitator to critique the event, summarize the participant evaluations, and assess how well the participants attained the outlined learning goals. It is also appropriate for the facilitator to identify any unmet or newly recognized learning needs and to make recommendations for follow-up activities and programs.

Examples of Structured Learning Activities

The following structured learning activities are offered as examples of ones that can be used as a component of a biomedical ethics education program.

Body Disposal

Goals:

1. Provide an opportunity for participants to explore personal desires concerning disposal of their earthly remains.
2. Allow participants to explore different social, religious, and cultural views concerning body disposal.
3. Encourage discussion of similarities and differences between group participants.

Categories:

Communication
Death and dying
Personal awareness
Values clarification

Group size: 25 to 30 participants

Minimum time: 60 minutes

Supplies:

- One copy of the "Body Disposal Handout" for each participant
- A writing instrument for each participant

Procedure:

1. As facilitator, introduce the activity to the learning group by explaining that the group will examine various options concerning the disposal of human remains after death.
2. Give each participant a copy of the "Body Disposal Handout" and tell them to take approximately five minutes to think about their personal choices and to fill out the form.
3. After all forms are completed, divide the learning group into four or five small groups and instruct each group to discuss the choices of the group members. (30 minutes)
4. Ask group members to focus on the religious, cultural, and social factors that influenced their selections.
5. At the conclusion of the small-group discussions, reconvene the learning group and use the following questions to stimulate large-group interaction.

Discussion:

1. What were your feelings as you considered each option?
2. What do you think that your family members would say about your choices? Would they be surprised?
3. Have you made these choices known to anyone previously? Will you now do so?
4. Do other members of your family have the same desires as you do? If not, why are there differences?
5. How will what you learned from this activity benefit you in your job?

Body Disposal Handout

Instructions: On this form, indicate the likelihood of whether you would choose the specified option concerning disposal of your body after death.

	Probable	Possible	Unlikely
Buried in family plot	______	______	______
Buried far from family	______	______	______
Cremated and ashes kept by family	______	______	______
Cremated and ashes buried	______	______	______
Cremated and ashes scattered	______	______	______
Body donated to science	______	______	______

Children's Hour

Goals:

1. Increase participant awareness of death-related influences from their childhood.
2. Explore the positive and negative aspects of exposing children to death.
3. Provide a forum for dialogue about death in terms of fantasy life.

Categories: Death and dying
Personal awareness

Group size: 25 to 30 participants

Minimum time: 60 minutes

Supplies:

- Flip chart and felt-tip markers
- A self-adhesive notepad (3 × 5) and a marker for each small group
- Tape
- A room large enough for the facilitator to hang several flip chart pages on a wall

Procedure:

1. Divide the learning group into several smaller groups of five or six individuals. Each group selects a discussion leader.
2. Instruct the small groups to think of as many book titles, stories, and fairy tales as they can remember from their childhood that contain a death or have a death-related theme (for example, *The Three Little Pigs, Bambi, Charlotte's Web*). (15 to 20 minutes)
3. Ask the discussion leader to write each title on a self-adhesive notepad sheet—one title per page.
4. Briefly reconvene the large group (small groups can remain in their places) and ask members to identify any apparent themes of the literature mentioned (for example, death of an enemy, death of a parent, terminal illness).
5. Write each theme on the flip chart—one per page—and tape the pages to a wall.
6. When all of the themes have been identified, the small groups regather to classify the titles, which they had previously listed, into one of these themes.
7. Instruct groups to place their self-adhesive notes on the flip chart page that represents the theme of their titles.
8. When all of the titles have been placed on the flip chart pages, lead a large-group discussion using the following questions.

Discussion:

1. Were you surprised at the number of titles that were identified? At the kinds of themes?
2. Why do you believe that children's stories contain so many references to death?
3. What other things may have an impact on childhood memories of death?
4. How does exposure to death and death-related themes at an early age influence how children deal with these issues?
5. At what age or developmental stage do you feel that children can begin to understand the differences between fact, fiction, and fantasy in relation to death-related information?
6. How can adults help children learn to cope with these issues?
7. What did you learn from this exercise? How will it benefit you in your job?

Death Journal

Goals:

1. Help participants identify various sources of information that may influence modern perceptions about death.
2. Create an understanding of the impact of the mass media on personal values.
3. Provide an opportunity for self-analysis concerning perceptions of death-related issues.

Categories: Death and dying
Personal awareness
Values clarification

Group size: 30 participants

Minimum time: Two sessions: Introductory session—15 minutes. Discussion session—90 minutes.

Supplies:

- Paper and a writing instrument for each participant
- Flip chart and felt-tip markers

Procedure: *Introductory session:*

1. Explain to the participants that they will be doing research at home to learn about the influence of the mass media on modern perceptions of death.
2. Ask the learning group members to select one of the following: television news, radio news, prime-time dramatic television shows, talk shows, or television cartoons. At home they are to spend two hours watching or listening to programs in their chosen category. They are to list every mention of death that occurs during that time. Group members should keep track of who or what died, how the death occurred, and why it happened.

Discussion session:

3. When the group later reconvenes for the discussion, ask the group members to share what they learned. Note information on the flip chart using graphs or lists.
4. Conduct a discussion using the following questions.

Discussion:

1. What did you learn about the volume of death-related subject matter that is covered in the media?
2. What are some of the ways in which our perceptions of death are influenced by the entertainment industry and by the news media?
3. What did you learn about people who produce news and entertainment shows with regard to their attitudes toward death and death-related themes?
4. How do you think that these attitudes affect the general public?
5. How is death generally portrayed in fictionalized settings? How is this different from real life?
6. What are the most frequent causes of death mentioned in the news? In the entertainment industry?
7. Do you think that the present type of media exposure has generally desensitized us all to the emotions surrounding death?
8. What influence does the media have on the development of values and personal ethics?
9. Did you learn information from this activity that will be useful to you at work?

First Death

Goals:

1. Assist participants to gain an understanding of how early exposure to death has influenced values and perceptions as an adult.
2. Identify early issues of honesty and trust.
3. Help participants identify unresolved issues related to terminal illness and death.

Categories: Communication
Death and dying
Personal awareness
Terminal/chronic illness

Group size: 25 to 30 participants

Minimum time: 45 to 60 minutes

Supplies: None

Procedure:

1. Begin the activity by explaining that many adult feelings and perceptions have their roots in early childhood experiences. This activity will help participants to identify early experiences that may have been influential in their personal development.
2. Ask the group members to close their eyes and to think back to their childhood. Tell them to try to remember the first significant death in their life. This may be the death of a grandparent or a pet or a memory of a death from film or television.
3. Ask the group members to remember as many details as they can about the experience. Remain quiet for two or three minutes as they think.
4. Divide the group into pairs and ask each person to discuss their death remembrances with their partner. Participants should focus on facts, feelings, and reactions. Give each person sufficient time to talk. (approximately 15 minutes total)
5. Reconvene the learning group and lead a discussion using the following questions.

Discussion:

1. What difficulties did you have in thinking about these early memories?
2. Did this activity raise any hidden emotions?
3. As you remembered your early experience, do you remember that the significant information about this death was given to you honestly, or were the facts hidden or distorted to "protect" you? Why do you think this was so?
4. How did the response of others at that time affect you in later years?
5. What have you done differently with or for your children as a result of your own early experiences of death?
6. How can adults help children deal with these issues?
7. How will what you learned from this activity help you to do your job differently?

Five Senses . . . Four . . . Three . . . Two . . . One . . .

Goals:

1. Enhance sensory awareness.
2. Provide participants with a greater understanding of their physical selves.
3. Develop an appreciation for the sensory limitations experienced by individuals who are chronically or terminally ill.

Categories: Personal awareness
Terminal/chronic illness

Group size: 15 to 20 participants

Minimum time: 60 to 90 minutes

Supplies:

- Each participant will need:
  —Earplugs
  —A blindfold
  —Nose clips
  —A pillow
- Popcorn and a popcorn popper
- 15 to 20 small paper cups
- Two pot lids or a large bell
- A room large enough for all the participants to spread out on the floor without touching anyone else

Procedure:

1. Explain to the group members that this activity is designed to provide them with an experience that will help them to understand some aspects of the type of sensory limitations often experienced by terminally or chronically ill individuals. Warn participants to expect surprises. Assure them that nothing harmful will take place.
2. Give each participant a blindfold, ear and nose plugs, and a pillow. Tell them to find a place on the floor where they will later be able to lie down without touching anything or anyone else.
3. As the participants are finding their spots, turn on the popcorn machine and allow the corn to begin to pop. After one or two minutes, instruct the participants to put on their nose plugs.
4. Distribute a small cup of the popped corn to each participant and tell the group to "enjoy the snack."
5. After the participants eat the popcorn, instruct them to put on their blindfolds, lie down with their heads on their pillows, relax, and get comfortable.
6. After about three minutes, make a loud noise by banging the pot lids or ringing the bell.
7. A minute or so later, inform the participants that the rest of the activity will take approximately 10 to 15 minutes and that they are to relax and rest until the activity is over. They may not, however, move at all once they are told to put their earplugs in. Inform them that while they are resting some of them will be touched, poked, and moved, but not in harmful ways. Tell participants that when they feel a tap on the top of their head, the activity is over and that they should remove all of the items and return to their seats. Ask the

participants to put in their ear plugs. Then proceed to touch, poke, and move some of the participants throughout the rest period.

8. Lead the following discussion.

Discussion:

1. What was your general reaction to this activity?
2. What was your feeling about the loss of your vision? Your hearing? Your ability to smell? Your freedom to move?
3. How did wearing a nose plug change your ability to taste? Did it alter your ability to enjoy the popcorn?
4. What was your reaction to the noise? After you heard it the first time, did you expect it again?
5. How did your sensory deprivation affect your ability to think clearly?
6. What was it like for you to wait to be touched, not knowing when—or if—it would happen?
7. How did you feel if you were touched?
8. How did you feel when the activity concluded and you were able to use all of your senses?
9. How did this activity change your perceptions concerning the sensory deprivation that may be a factor in the lives of ill patients?

Good Death—Bad Death

Goals:

1. Provide participants with an opportunity to clarify their own beliefs about terminal illness and death and dying.
2. Explore a form of nonverbal expression.
3. Increase awareness of individual philosophies concerning end-of-life issues.

Categories:

Communication
Death and dying
Personal awareness
Terminal/chronic illness
Values clarification

Group size: 10 to 15 participants

Minimum time: 60 to 90 minutes

Supplies:

- Two large sheets of drawing paper and a box of crayons for each participant
- Masking tape
- A room large enough to display all artwork on the walls

Procedure:

1. Give each participant two large sheets of paper and a box of crayons. Tell them to label one sheet "Good Death" and the other "Bad Death."
2. Tell the participants that they have 40 minutes to draw whatever they would like to depict the labels on their sheets.
3. Remind participants that artistic ability is not a prerequisite for this activity. Say that they can express themselves through colors, symbols, or realistic representations but may not use words.
4. After all of the pictures have been completed, hang them on the walls. Invite the entire group to look at all of the drawings.
5. Ask each group member to select one of the drawings that is not his or her own and to interpret it for the group.
6. After everyone has had an opportunity to discuss one of the drawings, lead the following discussion.

Discussion:

1. What was the experience of using nonverbal expression like for you?
2. What symbols were used in the group's drawings?
3. What common themes were expressed?
4. Did the other group member interpret your drawing as you expected or intended?
5. How did seeing all of the pictures displayed make you feel?
6. What can be learned about an individual's values and beliefs through this activity?
7. What did you learn about yourself through this activity? Can anything that you learned help you in your job?

Highs and Lows of Life

Goals:

1. Assist participants to identify meaningful events in their lives that have influenced how they currently view difficult issues.
2. Foster understanding of the development of personal perceptions.
3. Provide a creative way for individuals to analyze personal historical events.

Categories: Communication
Personal awareness
Values clarification

Group size: 20 to 25 participants

Minimum time: 60 minutes

Supplies:

- One copy of the "Highs and Lows of Life Handout" for each participant
- A large sheet of paper and a writing instrument for each participant

Procedure:

1. Distribute the handout and other supplies to each participant.
2. Explain to the group that everyone has had many experiences in life that have influenced one's ability to handle difficult situations. This activity is designed to help the participants identify the specific events that have been critical in their own lives.
3. Ask the participants to follow directions on the handout and to make a graph of the most significant events that they can remember. These events can include a birth, a death, graduation from college, or a special trip or other event. Encourage participants to be specific. The events can be positive or negative, and there is no number required in either category. Participants also are to write the date of each event and put the events in chronological order on the graph.
4. Allow participants 40 minutes to complete their graph. Then lead the discussion.

Discussion:

1. What did you learn about yourself through this activity?
2. What difficulty did you have in identifying particular events?
3. Were you surprised at the number of high or low points that you identified?
4. What emotions were evoked as you remembered these events?
5. What patterns did you identify in the events that you identified? What does this tell you?
6. As you did this activity, did you become aware of events that you would probably include if you were to do the activity 10 to 20 years from now?

Highs and Lows of Life Handout

Instructions: Transfer the form below to the large sheet of paper you were given. Use that form to make a line graph of the significant events in your life. Label each event at the bottom of the graph, indicate the year that the event occurred, and place the event either at a high point or low point on the chart, depending on how you felt about the experience.

Most wonderful

Average

Most terrible

Year (event)

Ethics for Everyone: A Practical Guide to Interdisciplinary Biomedical Ethics Education.

If I Could Control the End of My Life . . .

Goals:

1. Encourage participants to explore personal mortality and end-of-life issues.
2. Encourage self-disclosure.
3. Provide an opportunity to analyze how difficult choices are made.

Categories:

Communication
Death and dying
Personal awareness
Terminal/chronic illness
Values clarification

Group size: 20 to 25 participants

Minimum time: 60 minutes

Supplies:

- One copy of "If I Could Control the End of My Life . . . Handout" for each participant
- A writing instrument for each participant

Procedure:

1. Explain that the experience is designed to open discussion and reflection on personal mortality and on end-of-life issues.
2. Give a copy of the handout and a writing instrument to each participant and instruct them to spend 5 to 10 minutes completing the form.
3. Divide the learning group into groups of two to three participants and ask them to share why they made their individual choices.
4. At the end of 30 minutes, reconvene the group and lead the debriefing discussion.

Discussion:

1. What were the common factors that influenced individual choices?
2. What is the influence of society and religion over these types of preferences?
3. What questions were most difficult to answer? Why?
4. What were your feelings knowing that, in reality, people would ultimately be unable to have any control over most of these factors?
5. What other things would you like to have control of at the end of your life?

If I Could Control the End of My Life . . . Handout

Instructions: Take a few moments to think about what you would want to happen at the end of your life. Fill in the blanks on this form with the answers that you believe are true for you.

- I want to die when I am ______________ years old.
- I hope my mate dies (circle one) before/after me.
- I would prefer to die of ______________ (event/disease).
- When I die I want to be (check one):

  _____ Alone

  _____ With my mate

  _____ With my whole family

  _____ With a health professional
- It's important for me to live at least until ______________.
- I (circle one) do/do not want to be aware that I am going to die.
- I want to be (check one):

  _____ Awake and alert until the last moment

  _____ Peacefully unconscious at the end

I'm Terminally Ill

Goals:

1. Provide participants with an opportunity to gain insight into their current significant relationships.
2. Examine communication styles.
3. Explore how different individuals cope with pressure and adversity.

Categories: Communication
Death and dying
Personal awareness
Terminal/chronic illness

Group size: Unlimited

Minimum time: 45 to 60 minutes

Supplies: None

Procedure:

1. Divide the learning group into small groups of no more than four individuals.
2. Ask the group members to pretend that they have each just been told that they have a terminal illness and have only a few months to live.
3. The group is to discuss:
   —Whom they would tell
   —Whom they would *not* tell
   —How they think this information would be told
   —How they believe that they would feel in this situation
4. After 20 to 30 minutes, reconvene the learning group for discussion.

Discussion:

1. What difficulties were there in deciding whom you would tell of your terminal illness?
2. What criteria did you use to decide to tell certain people but to keep the information from others? Were all these criteria logical?
3. What methods were used to tell people about the illness?
4. What emotions did this experience generate?
5. How could someone prepare if he or she really had to tell someone that you were terminally ill?
6. Would you want to know if people in your life were terminally ill?
7. How can information you learned from this activity be used in a health care setting?

Living Will

Goals:

1. Enable participants to examine personal choices concerning end-of-life decisions.
2. Gain insight into various approaches to end-of-life choices.
3. Identify personal issues that may not have been previously addressed.

Categories:
Death and dying
Personal awareness
Terminal/chronic illness
Values clarification

Group size: 25 to 30 participants

Minimum time: 60 to 120 minutes

Supplies:

- One copy of "Living Will Handout" (or other version of a living will) for each participant
- A writing instrument for each participant

Procedure:

1. Introduce the activity by explaining the purpose and uses of a living will. (See chapter 3.)
2. Distribute the supplies to each participant, with instructions to complete the handout in approximately 10 minutes.
3. After the participants have completed the handout, lead the discussion.

Discussion:

1. How did you feel about this activity?
2. What things that you had not previously considered did the experience make you aware of?
3. Were you surprised at any of the choices you made?
4. Do you believe that a living will is an important document for everyone to complete? Why or why not?
5. What actions might you take as a result of participating in this activity?

Living Will Handout

I, ______________, being of sound mind, willfully and voluntarily make this declaration to be followed if I cannot make or communicate decisions about my medical care. Those around me should rely on this document for instructions about measures that could keep me alive. This declaration reflects my firm commitment to refuse life-sustaining treatment under the circumstances indicated below.

My attending physician should withhold or withdraw life-sustaining treatment that serves only to prolong the process of my dying if I should be in a terminally ill condition or in a state of permanent unconsciousness.

Treatment should be limited to measures to keep me comfortable and to relieve pain, including any pain that might occur by withholding or withdrawing life-sustaining treatment.

In addition, if I am in a terminally ill condition or a state of permanent unconsciousness, I feel especially strong about the following treatments:

I ______ DO ______ DO NOT want cardiac resuscitation

I ______ DO ______ DO NOT want blood or blood products

I ______ DO ______ DO NOT want tube feeding or any other artificial or invasive form of nutrition (food) or hydration (water)

I ______ DO ______ DO NOT want mechanical respiration (artificial breathing)

I ______ DO ______ DO NOT want kidney dialysis

I ______ DO ______ DO NOT want antibiotics

I ______ DO ______ DO NOT want any form of surgery or invasive diagnostic tests

I realize that if I do not specifically indicate my preference regarding any of the forms of treatment listed above, I may receive that form of treatment.

Extra instructions: Following are instructions about any special fears or desires.

Other Instructions:

I ______ DO ______ DO NOT want to designate another person as my surrogate to make medical treatment decisions for me if I should be incompetent and in a terminally ill condition or in a state of permanent unconsciousness.

Name of surrogate (if applicable) ______________________________________

Address ____

____

This declaration was made on ________________ (date). I have thought about this advance directive carefully. I know what it means and want to sign it. I have chosen two witnesses, neither of whom is a member of my family, nor will inherit from me when I die.

____

Declarant's signature

____

Witness's signature

____

Witness's signature

My Fears

Goals:

1. Help participants identify personal fears.
2. Discover similarities and differences between group members.
3. Encourage self-disclosure.

Categories: Personal awareness
Values clarification

Group size: 25 to 30 participants

Minimum time: 60 minutes

Supplies:

- A supply of self-adhesive note papers and a felt-tip marker for each participant
- Four to six large sheets of newsprint for each pair
- A room where all the newsprint sheets can be placed on the walls at the same time

Procedure:

1. Give each participant in the learning group a supply of self-adhesive note paper and a marker. Instruct them to take five minutes to write down everything that they can think of that they fear (one fear per sheet).
2. Ask the participants to form pairs and to trade their stack of note papers with their partner. Give sheets of newsprint to each pair.
3. Ask the participants to take their partner's fears and to group them into categories, such as fears related to personal safety, fears related to the future, fears about the environment or fears of the unknown. The self-adhesive sheets from each category are put on a separate sheet of newsprint, which is labeled with the title of the category. (10 minutes)
4. Pairs are to discuss what they learned about each other from the information in the categories and to also compare their similarities and differences concerning categories or specific fears. (15 minutes)
5. The final step in this activity before the discussion phase is to hang all of the large sheets of newsprint on the walls of the room, also grouping them by categories.

Discussion:

1. How did this experience make you feel?
2. How alike or dissimilar are your fears compared with those of your partner? Compared with others in the group?
3. What were the common themes or fears that were identified?
4. In your opinion, were all the fears that were identified reasonable, or did some not make any sense to you?
5. To what degree do personal experiences, lifestyles, values, and backgrounds affect our fears?
6. Which of your fears was the most significant for you? Why?
7. Was there anything that you learned from this activity that could be used in your work setting?

My Last Hour

Goals:

1. Increase awareness of personal mortality.
2. Provide an opportunity for participants to assess present relationships.
3. Encourage self-evaluation.

Categories:
Death and dying
Personal awareness
Terminal/chronic illness
Values clarification

Group size: 10 to 15 participants

Minimum time: 90 minutes

Supplies:

- Two pillows for each participant
- A room large enough for participants to lie on the floor without touching each other
- Facial tissues

Procedure:

1. Instruct participants to find a place on the floor where they can lie comfortably on their backs without touching any other group member. Give each participant two pillows, one to put under their head and the other for under their knees.
2. Dim the lights.
3. Explain that the group will be participating in a guided imagery activity. The participants will be given general instructions, and they are to use their own imaginations to place themselves into the story.
4. Tell the participants that some individuals will find this exercise easy to do and others may find it extremely difficult. The focus of the exercise is inward, and everyone should thus participate in the way and to the degree that is most comfortable for that individual.
5. Read the following instructions aloud:

> Make yourself as comfortable as possible. Lie with your arms at your sides and your legs uncrossed. Keep your eyes closed and your body still.
>
> Relax and let the worries and the troubles of your real world float away. Feel the places in your body where there is tension. Relax them. Feel the warmth of your muscles. Feel the peacefulness around you. Take a few deep breaths. Hold them. Then let them out slowly. (*pause*)
>
> Open your mind and your imagination. Listen to my voice and allow your thoughts to flow freely. (*pause*)
>
> Imagine that you are at the end of your life. You have been ill for a very long time. You know that the end is near, and although you are sad, you are ready to let go. You have lost your ability to communicate and to move but you are aware of your surroundings. (*pause*)
>
> Picture the room where you are. Are you in a hospital? A nursing home? At home in your own bed? (*pause*) What can you see in this room? Are there mementos of your life? (*pause*) Photos of loved ones? Are there machines and monitors? What sounds do you hear? (*pause*)
>
> Look at the people who are with you. Who is in the room? (*pause*) Is your mate there? Your children? Your friends? Professional health care workers? (*pause*) How do these people feel? What are they saying to you? (*pause*) What would you say to them if you were able to speak? (*pause*)

Who is missing from the people who are with you? Is there someone with whom you have had a problem? An argument? (*pause*) Does that person know you are dying? If that person had been aware that you were ill, would the person have been able to resolve your problem? What would you say to that person if you could have a conversation now? (*pause*)

Someone has come to pray for you. Who is this person? Are your religious beliefs strong? Does this visit bring you comfort? What do you believe will happen to you when you leave this life? Where are you going? What will it be like? (*pause*)

Your heart begins to beat more slowly. Your breaths are further and further apart. You can no longer see. Your hearing is fading. You can feel someone touching you, holding your hand. You can barely hear the words that they whisper. (*pause*)

And now you have died. Your soul has left your body and is floating above the bed. What do you see? (*pause*) What do you hear? (*pause*) How do you feel? (*pause*) What has been the reaction of the people in the room?

As you float away you watch the scene below you fade away. Your death is complete. (*long pause*)

When you are ready, slowly come back into your living body. Take a few deep breaths. Move your arms and legs. Open your eyes. Sit up and return to your seat.

6. Conduct the following discussion.

Discussion:

1. What was it like for you to imagine your death? What was your emotional response to this experience?
2. Did you experience anything that disturbed you?
3. Which moments did you find comforting?
4. Were there any aspects that you could not allow yourself to fully experience?
5. Did you learn anything new about your preferences concerning your death?
6. Did you find any aspect of the experience humorous? Why?
7. What did you learn about your relationships with the people whom you envisioned were by your side at the end?
8. What feelings did you experience as you envisioned your soul leaving the room?
9. How has this experience changed you?

Obituary

Goals:

1. Assist participants to identify diversity in comfort levels with death issues.
2. Facilitate an understanding of societal norms concerning death issues.
3. Encourage self-expression.

Categories: Death and dying
Personal awareness

Group size: 20 participants

Minimum time: 60 minutes

Supplies:

- A sheet of paper and a writing instrument for each participant
- The obituary section of several different newspapers—one section for each participant

Procedure:

1. Distribute the supplies to the participants and ask them to take about five minutes to review the newspaper obituaries.
2. Lead a discussion concerning the type of information that usually is contained in an obituary and the differences between styles of obituaries (for example, between an obituary in the hometown paper and one in the *New York Times*).
3. Tell each group member to select one individual whom they know well (not a close family member) and to write an obituary for that individual. (15 minutes)
4. After the obituaries are completed, ask participants to read them to the group.
5. Lead the discussion.

Discussion:

1. What did it feel like to write an obituary about someone else? How did you feel when you read it aloud?
2. How did you approach this assignment? What information did you consider including or excluding? On what did you base your final decision?
3. What are your feelings concerning the inclusion in an obituary of specific details, such as the length of illness; the cause of death; or the name of the unmarried partner of the deceased.
4. What do obituaries tell us about the values, beliefs, and opinions of an individual or of society?

Rank Order

Goals:

1. Help promote self-awareness.
2. Encourage self-disclosure.
3. Help participants identify personal feelings, values, and beliefs.

Categories: Personal awareness
Values clarification

Group size: 25 to 30 participants

Minimum time: 60 to 90 minutes

Supplies:

- Two copies of the "Rank Order Handout" for each participant
- A writing instrument for each participant

Procedure:

1. Explain that this activity is designed to expose participants to the diversity of values that are found in any group of individuals. It is intended to open discussion on belief systems and to help group members identify and name some of their personal values.
2. Distribute the supplies and ask the participants to take five minutes to complete one copy of the handout.
3. After the handouts are completed, divide the learning group into groups of four or five individuals.
4. Ask the small groups to discuss their choices and to try to convince the other group members that their choices are the "correct" ones. (15 to 20 minutes)
5. After the small groups have concluded their discussions, ask the participants to complete the second copy of their handout without looking at the first one.
6. Reconvene the learning group and lead the discussion.

Discussion:

1. What made this activity easy or difficult?
2. What emotions did you experience while doing the activity?
3. How did you feel about having your beliefs challenged?
4. How did your second ranking compare with the first one? What convinced you to make any changes when you did the ranking the second time?
5. What items would you have added to (or deleted from) the lists?
6. What did you learn from this activity? Can any of what you learned be used in the work setting?

Rank Order Handout

Instructions: Look at the list below. Rank each of the items on the list from 1 to 10 according to the indicated scale.

Scale: 10 = most important
1 = least important

______ Wealth
______ Good health
______ A long life (until 100 years old)
______ Job satisfaction
______ A happy marriage
______ Numerous friendships
______ Fame
______ Philanthropy
______ Community involvement
______ Creativity

Ethics for Everyone: A Practical Guide to Interdisciplinary Biomedical Ethics Education.

Religious Influence

Goals:

1. Help participants to discover the origins of their ethical beliefs.
2. Provide an opportunity to gain insight into various value systems.
3. Identify similarities and differences among different faiths.

Categories: Personal awareness
Values clarification

Group size: 25 to 30 participants

Minimum time: 60 minutes

Supplies: None

Procedure:

1. Ask participants to reflect on their religious background and upbringing and to think about the influence that religion has had on their approach to illness, death and dying, and decision making.
2. Divide the learning group into several groups of four or five participants. (The small groups should be as religiously diverse as possible.)
3. Ask the small groups to discuss (for about 45 minutes) what they know about the teachings of their religion or denomination concerning:
   - Life support
   - Ordinary/extraordinary care
   - Termination of treatment
   - Assisted suicide
   - Organ and tissue donation
   - Body disposal and funeral customs
4. Reconvene the learning group and lead the discussion.

Discussion:

1. What were the similarities and differences in the beliefs that were discussed?
2. What questions did this discussion raise about the teachings of your faith? Did you know the position of your religion concerning each of these subjects, or are there areas about which you have questions?
3. What did you learn about the beliefs of other faiths that surprised you?
4. How do you think that your personal religious training influenced your present beliefs and practices? Have there been any changes since you have become an adult?
5. How was this discussion beneficial to you?
6. Is your religion (or religion in general) as important to you now as it was 10 or 20 years ago?
7. What information from this discussion would be useful to workers in a health care setting?

Remember Me

Goals:

1. Help participants come to terms with their own mortality.
2. Provide an opportunity to assess personal accomplishments.
3. Stimulate self-analysis.

Categories: Death and dying
Personal awareness
Values clarification

Group size: 20 to 25 participants

Minimum time: 90 minutes

Supplies: Paper and a writing instrument for each participant

Procedure:

1. Explain that participants will be conducting an exercise in self-reflection and self-analysis and that they should be as introspective, truthful, and objective as possible.
2. Distribute the supplies and give the group one hour to do the following:

   Identify the individual who would be most likely to give the eulogy at your funeral if you were to die today. Write the eulogy that you believe that individual would give on your behalf.

3. At the end of the hour, ask any participants who are willing to read their eulogies to the learning group.
4. When all of the eulogies have been read, lead the discussion.

Discussion:

1. What was your first reaction to being told to write about yourself as others see you?
2. Was this assignment easy or difficult for you? Why?
3. What did you discover about yourself as you wrote? Did you learn anything about your personal values or beliefs?
4. Did you emphasize (or eliminate) any aspect of your life?
5. How difficult was it to share your eulogy with the group? (For those who did not read their eulogy aloud, why not?)
6. How did you feel hearing the eulogies of others in the group?

Sudden Death

Goals:

1. Help participants to focus on feelings related to the unpredictability of death.
2. Promote awareness of personal coping styles.
3. Encourage self-disclosure.

Categories: Communication
Death and dying
Personal awareness

Group size: Unlimited

Minimum time: 45 to 60 minutes

Supplies: Paper and a writing instrument for each participant

Procedure:

1. Divide the learning group into pairs.
2. Give participants a sheet of paper and a writing instrument and tell them to write the names of the 10 most important people in their lives.
3. Ask a group member to select a number from 1 to 10.
4. Tell the group members to find the name on their list that corresponds to that number and to cross off the name. Next to it, they are to write "deceased" and today's date.
5. Instruct the pairs to discuss their feelings about the "loss" of that individual in their lives.
6. After 10 minutes, ask the group to form new pairs. Tell the group to cross off the first name on their list and to also label that person as deceased. (Note: If the first number selected was the number 1, ask the group to cross off the last name on the list.)
7. The new pairs then discuss their feelings concerning this "loss." (10 minutes)
8. Reconvene the learning group for the discussion.

Discussion:

1. What were your reactions to crossing off the names on your lists?
2. How did your responses change from the first individual you "lost" to the second?
3. What emotions (for example, anger, sadness, fear) did you experience concerning the suddenness of your "loss"?
4. Did you experience a feeling of loss of control because the decision concerning who would "die" was arbitrary?
5. Will you react differently to the individuals who "died" in this exercise the next time you see them?

This Money Goes to . . .

Goals:

1. Help participants explore personal value systems.
2. Increase understanding of how personal beliefs influence decision making.
3. Offer insight into the complexities of a decision-making process.

Categories: Personal awareness
Values clarification

Group size: 25 to 30 participants

Minimum time: 60 minutes

Supplies:

- A copy of the "This Money Goes to . . . Handout" for each group
- A writing instrument for each group

Procedure:

1. Explain that this activity will enable participants to explore their own value systems and their strategies for decision making. It is also designed to compare and contrast the beliefs and value systems of others and to open a discussion on the differences that might affect how decisions are made.
2. Divide the learning group into groups of four to five participants.
3. Give each group one copy of the handout. The group is to decide collectively how to distribute the allocated funds. Each group is to select one individual to lead the discussion and to report the results to the large group.
4. Inform the participants that they are to use their powers of persuasion and reason to convince the other members of their group how to distribute the money.
5. After 30 to 40 minutes, reconvene the large group. The small-group leaders report their group's decisions and the rationale for their choices. A discussion follows.

Discussion:

1. How similar or different were the initial ideas for allocating the money among the members in your group?
2. Would your donation suggestions have been different if the amounts you gave away had been made public?
3. What would you have done differently if you had only $5,000 to donate? Or if you had to give all $5 million to only one organization?
4. How did personal values and your past history influence choices?
5. What other options would you have added to the list of possible recipients?

This Money Goes to . . . Handout

Instructions: Your committee is in charge of the distribution of $5 million. Your instructions are to use the money to do good works and to distribute it fairly. However, the distribution will be handled anonymously, and no one but your committee will know how the money was spent. Indicate how much of this money, if any, you would distribute in the following categories:

$ ________________ Buy new, much-needed equipment for the local community hospital

$ ________________ Conduct research on a deadly disease

$ ________________ Establish a program for children who are mentally retarded

$ ________________ Have the committee attend an excellent conference called "Using Donations Wisely"

$ ________________ Distribute free birth control devices to teenagers

$ ________________ Build a research facility to find a cure for the common cold

$ ________________ Establish an herbal medicine center

$ ________________ Provide a shelter for the large population of drug-using transients who have come to your town

Tombstone

Goals:

1. Help participants come to terms with their own mortality.
2. Offer an opportunity for self-analysis.
3. Promote self-disclosure.

Categories: Death and dying
Personal awareness
Values clarification

Group size: Unlimited

Minimum time: 60 minutes

Supplies:

- Paper and a box of crayons or felt-tip markers for each participant
- Tape
- A room with enough wall space for all drawings to be displayed at the same time

Procedure:

1. Distribute the supplies to the participants and instruct them to create a picture of the tombstone that they would like to have placed on their own grave. The drawings can be as creative or as simplistic as the participants choose. The tombstone should contain all of the essential information about the "deceased" as well as a 10- to 15-word epitaph. (15 minutes)
2. After the drawings are completed, the group members take turns explaining their creations to the rest of the group.
3. After the explanation, ask the group members to hang their tombstone on the wall to create a "group graveyard."
4. Lead the discussion.

Discussion:

1. What was this experience like for you? What emotions did it generate?
2. What problems did you have in deciding what to write?
3. Did you want to write more or less than you had space for? Why do you think this is so?
4. What was your reaction to the finished "group graveyard"?
5. Why do you think society uses tombstones? What purpose do they serve?
6. What have you learned from this activity?

What's Missing?

Goals:

1. Help participants develop an understanding of the role of various losses in their lives.
2. Encourage self-disclosure.
3. Increase awareness of internalized emotions.

Categories: Personal awareness
Values clarification

Group size: 20 to 25 participants

Minimum time: 60 minutes

Supplies: One large sheet of drawing paper and a box of crayons or felt-tip markers for each participant

Procedure:

1. Distribute the supplies to each participant and instruct them to divide the drawing paper into fourths.
2. Ask the participants to take a few minutes to reflect on the significant losses in their lives and to identify the four losses that were most difficult for them to cope with.
3. Instruct the participants to draw a picture of each of these losses in each of the fourths of the paper. (30 minutes)
4. When the drawings are complete, have group members take turns explaining their creations to the group.
5. Lead the group in the discussion.

Discussion:

1. Was it easy or difficult to identify specific losses in your life?
2. What emotions resurfaced as a result of this activity?
3. What categories of losses were most often identified by the group members?
4. How did the types of losses and the magnitude of those losses affect you over time?
5. Before this activity, how aware were you of the impact of nondeath losses on your life?
6. What would be the worst loss you could experience today?
7. What support and coping mechanisms have you developed to help you deal with losses?
8. What did you learn from this activity? How can that learning be applied to your work setting?

Who Decides?

Goals:

1. Help participants to develop an understanding of the loss of control experienced by people who are seriously ill.
2. Encourage reflection on personal choices.
3. Help develop an understanding of various personal needs.

Categories: Communication
Death and dying
Personal awareness
Terminal/chronic illness

Group size: 25 to 30 participants

Minimum time: 60 to 90 minutes

Supplies:

- Felt-tip markers and self-adhesive notepads for each small group (three)
- Flip chart paper
- Tape
- A room where several sheets of flip chart paper can be taped to the walls at the same time

Procedure:

1. Explain that the activity is designed to raise awareness of some of the difficulties that individuals face as they progress from a state of health to a state of serious illness.
2. Divide the learning group into three small groups. Each group selects a discussion leader and a recorder. Give each a self-adhesive notepad, a marker, and three sheets of flip chart paper. The small groups move to a place where the flip chart papers can be taped to a wall and viewed during the activity. The group recorder labels one of the flip chart papers "Healthy"; another "Ill"; and the third, "Dying."
3. Assign each group one of the following time periods:
   - Wake-up to noon (includes breakfast)
   - Noon to 5 p.m. (includes lunch)
   - 5 p.m. to bedtime (includes dinner)
4. Ask each group to brainstorm and to identify each decision that a healthy person might make during that time period (for example, what time to get up, what to wear, what to have for breakfast). The group recorder writes each decision on a separate sheet of the self-adhesive notepad and places the sheets on the flip chart paper labeled "Healthy." (15 minutes)
5. After all of the decisions have been placed on the flip chart paper, instruct the group leader to conduct a discussion concerning which of the decisions that the group identified would still be able to be made by an individual who was moderately ill. These self-adhesive sheets are then moved to the flip chart paper labeled "Ill." (10 minutes)
6. Instruct the group leader to lead the participants in a discussion that will identify which of the items on the "Ill" sheet would be decisions that could still be made by a person who was dying. These self-adhesive sheets are then moved to the last flip chart paper. (10 minutes)
7. After the small groups have finished their tasks, reconvene the learning group and lead the discussion.

Discussion:

1. What difficulty did you have in identifying all the choices that an individual might have to make during a particular time period?
2. What has this exercise taught you concerning how illness and disease affect an individual's ability to maintain control in his or her life?
3. What have you learned concerning your personal attitudes toward individual control and decision making?
4. What were your feelings as the choices began to be eliminated? How would you feel if you were the person who could no longer make these choices?
5. What differences would there be for someone who lost the ability to make choices because of an appendectomy, as opposed to someone who lost decision-making ability because of terminal cancer?
6. How important is it for patients to retain control in their lives?
7. How will this activity help you in your work?

Suggested Readings

Cooper, C. L., and Harrison, K. Designing and using group activities: variables and issues. In: J. W. Pfeiffer and J. J. Jones, editors. *The 1976 Annual Handbook for Group Facilitators.* La Jolla, CA: University Associates, 1976.

Forbess-Greene, S. *The Encyclopedia of Icebreakers.* San Diego: University Associates, 1983.

Knott, J. E., Ribar, M. C., Duson, B. M., and King, M. R. *Thanatopics: A Manual of Structured Learning Experiences for Death Education.* Kingston, RI: S.L.E. Publications, 1982.

Pfeiffer, J. W., editor. *The Encyclopedia of Group Activities.* San Diego: University Associates, 1989.

Training Directors Handbook. Waterford, CT: Prentice Hall, 1989.

Chapter Seven

Role Play

Role play, a type of structured learning activity, is uniquely suited to the teaching of interpersonal communication and human relations skills. It allows participants to use their intellectual knowledge and their cognitive understanding in practical and applied settings.

Role play gives participants an opportunity to practice skills by creating hypothetical scenarios that would be similar to situations that the participants may encounter either on the job or in their personal lives. These scenarios are realistic but not real. They therefore provide a safe environment in which the participants can explore various components of difficult issues while being supported by the learning environment. As such, role play is an ideal tool to use to assist health care workers to gain insight into biomedical ethics issues while exploring their own ethical beliefs and value systems. At the same time, the participants are exposed to the attitudes and beliefs of others and to the diverse coping mechanisms that other individuals may demonstrate.

As with all structured learning activities, role play should not be used in isolation. It should, instead, be used as part of a broader educational experience. Role play should follow—and be used as reinforcement for—a cognitive component such as a lecture, video discussion, or structured learning activity in which a particular content area or human relations skill has been addressed.

Steps to Conduct a Role Play

There are six basic steps to conducting a role play. These steps, discussed in more detail in the following subsections, are:

- Step 1: Introduction
- Step 2: Assignment of roles
- Step 3: Audience preparation
- Step 4: Enactment
- Step 5: Discussion
- Step 6: Follow-up

Step 1: Introduction

The first step in conducting a role play is for the facilitator to provide the learning group with an overview of role play in general and to give an explanation of how the current activity will proceed. A brief summary of the rationale for the role play and a synopsis of the problem that will be addressed should also be provided as well as an overview of the goals and learning objectives for the experience.

The introduction to a role play should be designed to help motivate the participants and minimize any anxiety they might be experiencing. It is common for adults to feel uncomfortable or embarrassed when they are asked to pretend, and this is especially true when they are asked to pretend in a role play that involves a difficult or emotionally stressful situation. Therefore, it is important for the facilitator to reinforce that acting ability is not a prerequisite to successful role play and that there is no right or wrong way for the participants to perform their roles. Participants should be informed that, in role play, learning will take place through doing, observing, self-analysis, or process discussions and that effective learning can take place either through positive reinforcement of something that has been done well or through the understanding of how something could have been done differently.

In addition, during the introduction to a role play that addresses biomedical ethics, death and dying, or terminal illness issues, it is important to alert participants to the possibility that the experience may evoke memories or intense and unexpected emotions, such as sadness, fear, anger, or grief. If participants are aware of this possibility and understand that such reactions are normal, they will be less likely to experience anxiety or concern if the emotions do surface.

Step 2: Assignment of Roles

After the entire learning group has been introduced to the role play, the facilitator selects the appropriate number of people for the role play and assigns a character role to each of those individuals (players). Each player is provided with a brief written synopsis of his or her character as well as with information about the situation in which the character is involved. Players may or may not be shown information about the other character roles.

The players are then asked to leave the room briefly to review their roles and to plan how they will play their parts. Players should be reminded not to discuss their role or their intended handling of that role with the other players.

Before the start of the actual role play, the facilitator meets with the players to clarify roles, if necessary, and to answer any questions. The facilitator reminds the players to remain in their character roles during the role play and encourages all members of the group to become actively involved in the discussion and in the process. The facilitator may also assist the group in deciding who goes first to open the role play.

Participants in the role play are encouraged to be creative but to remain realistic. They are also told that if the experience becomes too emotional or too difficult, they may ask for a break or for the activity to be stopped.

Step 3: Audience Preparation

While the individuals who will be acting as players are out of the room, the facilitator prepares the audience by giving them an overview of the characters who will be in the role play and by providing a synopsis of the situation in which the characters find themselves. The facilitator also distributes observation sheets to each member of the audience. (See figure 7-1.) These sheets are designed to help include all members of the learning group in the activity by providing them with a way to organize their thoughts and reactions to the experience. The information that audience members record on the observation sheets will be useful to them during the discussion period that follows the role play.

Step 4: Enactment

The enactment phase of a role play usually takes no longer than 10 to 15 minutes. Longer experiences may be appropriate if there are numerous characters in the play or if the interaction is particularly meaningful and relevant.

During the enactment, players assume the identity of the character role to which they have been assigned and discuss that character's situation as if it were real. While the role play is in progress, the audience members remain uninvolved and do not interact with the players. The audience members only observe the interactions and make notes on their observation sheets for later reference.

The facilitator also generally does not interact with the players while the role play is being enacted. However, there are times when intervention from the facilitator would be not only appropriate but necessary. For example:

- If one of the players monopolizes all the conversation and does not permit the other players to act out their roles
- If a player steps out of his or her character role and begins to respond personally
- If the role play begins to move too quickly or is not moving at all
- If the emotional level becomes too intense

In addition, it is frequently the facilitator who guides the players to conclude the role play either when the issues have been sufficiently addressed or when the allotted time has elapsed.

Figure 7-1. Sample Role Play Observation Sheet

Community Hospital
Hometown, PA

Role Play Observation Sheet

Which characters are taking the lead in the discussion?

How does each character make you feel?

What are the issues that are surfacing?

What is being handled well?

How could the conflicts be handled differently?

What emotional responses are being generated?

Did the group focus on the root of the problem?

What other positive and negative aspects of the issue could have been addressed?

What was your general reaction to this role play?

Ethics for Everyone: A Practical Guide to Interdisciplinary Biomedical Ethics Education.

Step 5: Discussion

Following the role play, the facilitator allows sufficient time for discussion so that both the players and the audience can process their reactions to and their feelings about the experience. Before the discussion, it is important for the facilitator to remind participants to be descriptive and not judgmental. Comments should be limited to *what* happened, not *why* it happened or who was responsible. In addition, discussion references should be made to character roles rather than to individual players (for example, "The patient said . . ." rather than "Mary said . . .").

The discussion occurs in two phases. In the first phase, the facilitator encourages the players to discuss their comfort levels with the role-playing process as well as their perceptions about what went well and what could have been handled differently. They are asked to express their feelings about the characters and the situation and to indicate whether they believe that the experience was meaningful for them. During the second phase, the audience members are asked to join in the discussion and to use the information from their observation sheets to comment on the process, the issues, and the interactions that occurred during the role play. At the conclusion of the discussion, there should be an opportunity for all members of the learning group to summarize how this role play might help them either on the job or in their personal lives.

Step 6: Follow-up

Because of the complex and sometimes distressing emotional responses that can occur in role plays dealing with biomedical ethics, death and dying, or terminal illness issues, there may be a need to provide participants (players or audience members) with additional follow-up discussion or supportive care after the conclusion of the educational experience. This need may exist for any member of the learning group, but it may be especially great for individuals for whom the role play evoked memories of actual difficult experiences, concerns about existing conflicts, or an awareness of unresolved personal issues. Therefore, during the role play, it is important for the facilitator to remain alert to the emotional responses that are being generated so that he or she can assist those in need to obtain follow-up support. This follow-up can be provided by the facilitator, if appropriate, or by someone else who is trained to deal with psychosocial and emotional issues, such as a member of the social services or pastoral care staff.

It should be noted that emotional responses to a role play may not occur during the actual educational event but may be delayed for several hours or even for days or weeks. As such, the availability of follow-up care should be ongoing and not time limited. Participants should be told of the possibility for the need for this type of service and should be made aware of how to access appropriate resources.

Role Play Variations

In addition to the structured single role play as just described, the following variations in the role-playing process can be used:

- Multiple role plays
- Role rotation
- Stop action

Multiple Role Plays

In this variation, the larger learning group is divided into several smaller groups. Using the same role play for each group, roles are assigned to each member of the smaller groups, with one member of the group assuming the role of observer/discussion leader. Only this individual will use the observation sheet. After the role play has been enacted, the observer/discussion leaders conduct the discussion for their own group.

Finally, the entire learning group reconvenes to discuss the experience and to compare and contrast how the role play evolved in each group. The observer/discussion leaders should take the lead in this aspect of the discussion; however, if time permits, all members of the groups should be encouraged to share their thoughts.

Role Rotation

In role rotation, each player in the role play group takes a turn at playing each of the character roles in the scenario. This enables the players to experience a variety of emotions, conflicts, and perspectives while permitting the observers to gain a more thorough understanding of the different ways a particular situation might develop. Role rotation can be used with either a structured single role play or multiple role plays.

Stop Action

In stop-action role play, the facilitator (who, as indicated previously, usually remains uninvolved in the action of the role play) breaks the action of the players at one or more strategic points in the role play and asks the players to comment on their feelings or reactions to what is happening. These specific stopping points cannot be predetermined and will depend on the perceptions of the facilitator and on the flow of the activity. The facilitator may choose to emphasize one dimension of what has transpired or may try to redirect the focus of the players to work on a particular skill or a specific aspect of one of the relationships being presented. Stop-action role play should be used judiciously and carefully, so as not to damage the flow of the action of the role play or to inhibit the involvement of the players with their character roles.

Sample Role Plays

The following role plays are examples of ones that could be used as a component of a biomedical ethics education program.

Role Play 1: Refusal to Accept Treatment

Patient: You are a 51-year-old man who has had kidney disease for the past four years. You have been able to function relatively normally during most of that period and have enjoyed an active lifestyle, which includes frequent travel, golf, and fishing. You have continued to work at your job as a marketing specialist, and until recently you had missed only a few days of work because of your illness.

During the last several weeks your health has deteriorated rapidly, and you have been off work most of that time. You have been depressed because you have been unable to maintain your active lifestyle. Your physician has previously discussed kidney dialysis with you on several occasions, and you have stated that you do not ever want "to be dependent on a machine." You have not changed your mind.

You are meeting with your physician, who has just informed you that your kidney function is deteriorating. If you do not begin dialysis immediately, you will die very soon.

Physician: You are the physician for a 51-year-old male patient who has very severe kidney disease. You have been treating this patient for the past four years and know that until recently he has continued to work and lead a very active lifestyle. You have discussed kidney dialysis with this patient in the past, but he has stated that he does not want "to be dependent on a machine." The patient's condition has deteriorated, and you have just informed him that if he does not start dialysis, he will die very soon.

You understand that the patient has the right to refuse this treatment. You believe, however, that he could adjust to the treatments and that, if he were to have dialysis, he could live a relatively normal life for many more years.

Role Play 2: Decisions Regarding a Level of Care

Husband: You are the husband of an 83-year-old woman who has advanced Alzheimer's disease. She is unable to provide self-care and does not recognize any of her family members. You and your children have provided care for your wife at home, and even though your relationship has changed drastically, you still love her deeply and want the best for her.

Your wife has been hospitalized after a stroke and she has contracted pneumonia. Her physician has asked to meet with you concerning the level of care that should be provided to your wife.

Physician: You are the physician for an 83-year-old woman who has Alzheimer's disease. She has been hospitalized after having a stroke and has contracted pneumonia. You have been giving her antibiotics, but they have not been successful in treating the pneumonia. Use of a stronger medication is an option. Although the patient has been cared for at home until now, you believe that if she survives the pneumonia she will require more care than the family can provide. You would recommend that the patient go into a nursing home.

You have asked to meet with the patient's husband in an effort to determine the level of treatment that should be provided to this patient. You believe that a do-not-resuscitate (DNR) order would be appropriate.

Role Play 3: Conflict of Values

Patient: You are a 78-year-old man who has lung cancer, which has spread to your bones and brain. You have been undergoing treatment for this disease for nine years. You have had radiation therapy and several courses of chemotherapy. You are ready to die and want all treatment stopped immediately. You have written a living will stating your wishes and have provided a copy to your wife and to your physician.

Wife: You are the wife of a 78-year-old man who has advanced cancer for which he has been treated for nine years. He has just given you a copy of a living will, which states that he wants to die. He wants all treatment stopped immediately. You are very confused and upset because this document goes against your and your husband's religious beliefs that "life should be preserved at all costs."

Adult child: You are the son of a 78-year-old man who has been battling cancer for the past nine years. You are aware that your father has decided that he wants all treatment stopped, and you support him in his decision. You are concerned, however, that your mother may try to go against his wishes because she believes that his judgment is affected by the cancer, which has spread to his brain. She has also stated to you that your father's request to die goes against his religious beliefs to "preserve life at all costs."

Chaplain: You are a hospital chaplain who has been asked to meet with a family concerning a patient's decision to stop treatment for advanced cancer. Your presence was requested because the patient's living will goes against his known religious beliefs about "preserving life at all costs."

Role Play 4: Termination of Treatment

Patient's sister: You are the sister of a 49-year-old woman who was severely beaten in a robbery. She has suffered massive brain damage and has been on a ventilator since her admission seven weeks ago. Your sister is unmarried and has no other relatives except your elderly parents, who live far away and are both in very poor health.

Your sister's physician has stated that there is "no hope" that the patient will ever be cured or that she will ever regain her former functioning level. He has given you the option of removing your sister from the machine and allowing her to die. You, however, believe in miracles and are not yet ready to give up hope that she will recover.

You have developed a relationship with one of the nurses who has been caring for your sister. You trust her and respect her judgment.

Physician: You are the physician for a 49-year-old woman who suffered massive brain damage from a beating. The patient's prognosis is grave, and you believe that keeping her on the ventilator is only delaying her death. You do not believe that there is any hope for a recovery.

The patient's elderly, ill parents live out of town, and you have been communicating with the patient's sister, who has very unrealistic expectations for her sister's chances of recovery. You have just suggested that it may be in the patient's best interest for the ventilator to be stopped. You are aware that the patient's sister has formed a positive relationship with one of the nurses in the unit.

Nurse: You are a nurse who has been caring for a 49-year-old woman who was severely beaten and who, as a result, has suffered massive brain damage. The patient's sister, to whom you have been providing a great deal of support, has been approached by the physician concerning the possibility of removal of the patient from the ventilator. The sister is expecting a miracle and does not want treatment stopped. You agree with the physician's assessment and believe that the treatment is futile. You walk in as the physician and the sister are discussing the situation.

Role Play 5: The Right to Know

Physician: You are the physician for a 78-year-old man who has a history of severe depression for which he has been hospitalized on numerous occasions. He has been taking a new medication, and for the last 18 months he has been mentally stable.

You have just received the results of a biopsy, which show that the patient has prostate cancer. You know that he has been terrified of getting cancer. You are aware that this is a very slow-growing cancer and that, given the patient's age, he will probably die of something other than the cancer. The patient is away on a fishing trip and has requested that you give the results of the tests to his wife.

Wife: You are the wife of a 78-year-old man who has a history of severe mental illness. You have spent many years watching him go in and out of mental hospitals. He has been on a new medication for 18 months and has been mentally well during that time.

You are meeting with your husband's physician, and you have just learned that your husband has prostate cancer. You do not want your husband to know about the cancer because you believe that the knowledge will cause a return of the mental illness. You have asked your husband's physician to tell your husband that he has a growth but not that the growth is malignant.

Adult child: You are the daughter of a 78-year-old man who has a history of mental illness. Your mother has asked you to meet with her and your father's physician to discuss the results of recent tests. You have just learned that the tests show that your father has prostate cancer. A decision needs to be made concerning what your father should be told about this illness. You believe that honesty is the best policy.

Role Play 6: Alternative Treatment

Patient: You are a 54-year-old woman who has always been somewhat of a back-to-nature specialist. You live with a male friend in a cabin in the woods, are a vegetarian, weave your own woolen cloth, and practice herbal medicine.

Your friend recently found you unconscious and took you to the hospital. Tests revealed that you are anemic and severely undernourished. You are angry that you have been hospitalized and want to go home so that you can begin to treat yourself with herbs.

Friend: You are the male companion of a 54-year-old woman who has been hospitalized for anemia and malnutrition. The patient shuns traditional medicine and wants you to take her home to your cabin in the woods. You are afraid that if she goes home, she will just get sicker, but you know that if you do not comply with her wishes, she will find a way to leave the hospital on her own.

Physician: You are the physician for a 54-year-old woman who is anemic and undernourished. She wants to be discharged so that she can return home and treat herself with nontraditional herbal medications. You know that if she leaves the hospital and does not get proper follow-up treatment, she will get sicker. You are considering a psychological evaluation to determine the patient's competency level.

Role Play 7: Between Parents and Child

Patient: You are a 14-year-old boy who has leukemia. You have been receiving treatment for more than a year but remain very ill and have been in and out of the hospital too many times to easily count. You have read a lot about the disease and know that people can die of leukemia. Recently, two of your friends, who had been hospitalized at the same time you were, died within a week of each other.

Your parents are always very happy around you and say you are "doing fine." You think they are lying to you. You have decided that, when you and your parents meet with your doctor, you are going to tell them that you want the whole truth.

Physician: You are the physician for a 14-year-old boy who is losing his battle with leukemia. His parents have demanded that you be optimistic around the child, but it is clear from the type of questions that the patient has been asking that he is beginning to grasp the seriousness of his condition.

Mother: You are the mother of a 14-year-old boy who has leukemia. You have watched him suffer through numerous treatments, all of which have been unsuccessful in arresting the progress of the disease. You have made every effort to be supportive and positive around your son, in the belief that he will do better if he has hope for a recovery.

You are firm in your belief that your son should not be told that he is going to die. You believe that such knowledge would serve no purpose, and you know that you would not be able to deal with the emotional strain that it would cause.

Father: Your 14-year-old son is dying of leukemia. The boy has not been told that his condition is terminal. Your wife has taken a firm stand that your son should be told only positive news and that the true extent of his illness should be kept from him. You have disagreed with this course of action from the beginning, but because of your wife's fragile emotional state, you have deferred to her wishes and have largely remained silent about your son's condition. Lately, however, your son has been asking probing questions and has seemed a bit more anxious than usual. You are beginning to wonder how much your son suspects.

Role Play 8: Friends Saying Goodbye

Patient: You are a 63-year-old woman who is in a home care hospice program. You are awake and alert, and your pain is under control. Your best friend has not been to visit you since a tearful visit while you were in the hospital several weeks ago. She calls often but is so upset over your illness that she has not been able to bring herself to visit face-to-face.

You have called your friend and requested that she come to see you. She has agreed, but you can tell she is apprehensive about confronting the fact that you are dying. You feel the need to reassure her and to say goodbye.

Friend: Your best friend since elementary school is dying. She is at home in a hospice program. You have wanted to visit her, but she looked so ill the last time you saw her in the hospital that all you did was cry when you looked at her. You have not wanted to upset her, so you have been calling rather than visiting.

Your friend has asked you to come to see her. You have agreed but, knowing that this will probably be the last time you see her alive, you are very apprehensive and concerned that you will not be able to keep your emotions in check. You plan to talk about anything except the fact that she is dying.

Role Play 9: Allocation of Resources

Physician: You are the physician for a 57-year-old man who has had a stroke. He is able to ambulate with minimal assistance and needs some help to eat, dress, and bathe himself. He is occasionally incontinent. The patient is alert and aware of his situation. He has been in the physical rehabilitation unit for several weeks and has made good progress. He has no communication difficulties. He is now ready for discharge from the hospital.

The patient's wife is refusing to take her husband home. She states that, even with the home care that will be available, she will not be able to provide for her husband's daily needs. She has requested that the patient remain in the hospital for several more weeks while she sees if she can arrange for a family member to move in to assist her. You do not believe that additional funds should be expended to provide hospital care for this patient.

Wife: You are the wife of a 57-year-old man who has had a stroke. He has made progress in his therapy over the last several weeks and his physician says that he is ready for discharge from the hospital. You do not want to take him home because you know that he will be very demanding and that you will be unable to provide for his care alone. Your husband has a history of being verbally and physically abusive, but you do not want to tell anyone about this unless you have no other choice. You want more time to try to get someone to move in to help you. You have asked your husband's physician to keep him in the rehabilitation unit until you can work things out.

Role Play 10: The Question of Suicide

Patient: You are a 36-year-old man with AIDS. You have decided that you do not want to die in the same way that you have seen many of your friends die, and you plan to commit suicide before you reach the last stages of your illness. You have asked your live-in companion to assist you in this endeavor.

Friend: You are the live-in companion of a 36-year-old man with AIDS. Your friend has told you that he has decided to kill himself rather than suffer through a long illness. You want to support him in this choice but are afraid of the legal implications.

Physician: Your 36-year-old patient with AIDS has asked you for a prescription for a sedative. You are surprised at this request because he has never indicated that he had problems sleeping.

You were concerned several months ago that this patient may have been suicidal; however, when you questioned him, he denied any thoughts of killing himself. You have decided to meet with the patient and his companion before prescribing the sedative.

Role Play 11: The Right to Die

Physician: Your patient is a 77-year-old man who has experienced a series of strokes and has diabetes and arthritis. He has been a widower for 35 years and lives with his daughter and her family. The patient is deeply religious and has told you many times that he is not afraid to die because he knows he will be united in heaven with his wife and with his God. He did not prepare a living will.

The patient had another stroke two days ago and is presently in a coma. He is unresponsive and unaware of his surroundings. It appears that this patient is dying.

Daughter: Your 77-year-old father has been hospitalized after having another stroke. His condition is obviously very serious, and you are unsure how much longer he can live.

You and your father have always been very close. He has lived with you since your mother's death 35 years ago, and you and he have shared many special times together. Although it is difficult for you to see your father in this condition, you are not yet ready to see him die. You have decided that you want all available technology used to prolong his life. You are going to ask your father's physician to provide your father with a full CODE if his heart should stop and to also provide him with artificial food and hydration.

Role Play 12: Organ and Tissue Transplantation

Physician: You are the physician for a 29-year-old woman who was brought to the emergency department after a near-fatal automobile accident. The patient was revived and placed on a ventilator, but neurological evaluations have shown that she is brain dead.

Husband: Your 29-year-old wife was involved in an automobile accident. She has been in the intensive care unit for the last 72 hours. Although her condition is obviously very critical and the doctor has explained to you that she is brain dead, you have been watching the machines and believe that she is still alive. You think that she might pull through.

Nurse: You have just been notified that a 29-year-old woman in the intensive care unit has been declared brain dead. As part of the hospital's transplant team, you are responsible for assisting the physician in approaching the patient's husband to determine if any of the woman's organs may be obtained for transplantation.

Role Play 13: Communication

Patient: You are an elderly patient who has been admitted to the hospital after a series of blackouts and falls. You have a fractured hip and a severely bruised left arm. You are not sure why you black out and fall so often, and the experiences really frighten you, but you are sure that your doctor will be able to make you well again.

Your doctor came to visit you earlier today and explained a variety of tests and procedures to you, none of which you understood. You did not, however, want to take up his valuable time, so you did not ask him any questions. After he left, you felt agitated and confused. You have been crying ever since.

Nurse: You just checked on an elderly patient and found her agitated and in tears. She explained that she does not understand what is happening to her or what her doctor just told her. She has asked you to "sort it all out." You volunteered to ask her doctor to come back, but the patient adamantly refused, saying that he had other patients to see.

Role Play 14: Decisions about Treatment Options

Patient: You are a 33-year-old, attractive, single woman who has just learned that she has a malignant lump in her breast. Your physician has offered you two options: (1) full removal of the breast with no follow-up chemotherapy or radiation or (2) lumpectomy (removal of only the mass) with both chemotherapy and radiation therapy after the surgery. You cannot decide which option to take and have asked your surgeon to help you choose. Your older sister, a breast cancer survivor, is going with you to talk to the surgeon.

Physician: Your patient, a 33-year-old woman with breast cancer, has been unable to choose between a mastectomy (without subsequent chemotherapy or radiation therapy) and a lumpectomy (followed by chemotherapy and radiation therapy). She has asked you to make a firm recommendation. You performed a mastectomy on the patient's older sister three years ago, and you are aware that this sister is encouraging your patient to have the lumpectomy.

Sister: You are the older sister of a patient who was recently diagnosed with breast cancer. You have also had the disease and underwent a mastectomy three years ago. Since the surgery, you have been depressed, your husband left you, and you lost your job. Although you had difficulty in these areas before your surgery, you are convinced that the mastectomy was the ultimate cause of your problems.

Your sister is seeing the same surgeon who treated you. On a recent visit to him, you shared your opinion concerning your sister's surgery and requested that he try to persuade your sister to have the lumpectomy.

Role Play 15: Closure

Physician: Your 81-year-old patient is dying. He has slipped into a coma and will probably die before morning. Your patient told you that he was not afraid to die but that he did not want to be alone when it happened.

Wife: You are the wife of an 81-year-old man who has just quietly and peacefully lapsed into a coma. He is dying. You have accepted his death and have said your goodbyes. You want to stay by his side until the end, but it is very difficult for you to watch, and you think you want to wait in the hall.

Son: Your father has just lapsed into a coma. Death will occur shortly. Your mother is having a very difficult time staying in the room with him for these final hours, and yet you believe that your father would want her there. You are much too upset to stay with him.

Grandson: You are at the hospital with your father and your grandmother. You are waiting for your grandfather to die. You are the oldest (and probably favorite) grandchild, and your relationship with your grandfather has been one of the most important relationships in your life. When he got sick, you promised him that you would stay with him until the end, and you intend to keep that promise. Even though he is in a coma, you believe that he can hear you, and you plan to tell him exactly how much he means to you. You do not, however, want to be alone with him at the end.

Chapter Eight

Case Studies

As indicated in chapter 4, it is important for individuals who are involved in a biomedical ethics education program to develop a knowledge of, and a comfort level with, a process that can be used for ethical thinking and reflection. An understanding of this process can be developed through practice, using discussion of actual or hypothetical cases in which there are ethical questions or ethical conflicts.

In many institutions, especially in the early phases of biomedical ethics education, there may be a reluctance to use actual (in-house) cases because of concerns about confidentiality, concerns about the willingness of staff to participate openly, or simply because of uncertainty related to the possible emotional impact that such discussions may generate. In these instances, hypothetical cases can be used in place of actual cases.

The case studies presented in this chapter can be used for this purpose. Although the people and events depicted in these scenarios are fictitious, each case represents a situation that, theoretically, could happen, and in which there are ethical issues that would need to be addressed. Additionally, each case offers variations that can be used to stimulate additional discussion. It is recommended that these cases be discussed in terms of a process for ethical thinking and reflection and that a form similar to the one depicted in figure 4-2 (p. 60) be provided to participants as a discussion guide.

The Case of Mr. A.

Mr. A. is a 31-year-old auto mechanic who lives at home with his wife, his 3-year-old daughter, and his father. Mr. A. has a loving relationship with his wife and has always been very close to his father. He has told many people that his father is his best friend. Father and son frequently hunt together on weekends. They play chess every evening and have been business partners for the last 11 years.

Recently Mr. A. was severely burned in a fire when an engine that his father had been repairing exploded at the shop. On the way to the hospital, Mr. A. told his father that the pain was so terrible that he wanted to die.

Mr. A.'s injuries are extensive. His face is severely disfigured, he has lost his vision in one eye and may lose vision in the other, both his hands had to be amputated, and he suffered second- and third-degree burns over more than 60 percent of the rest of his body. If Mr. A. survives, he will need years of extensive, costly therapy. Mr. A. is heavily medicated for pain and is unable to communicate with his family or caregivers.

Over the last 24 hours Mr. A. has developed a severe infection, and his physicians are suggesting a change in medication to combat this complication. Mr. A.'s father, however, has stated that he "can no longer watch the boy suffer." He feels that treatment should be stopped so that his son can die. He has told Mr. A.'s wife about her husband's request to die, but she feels that her husband was delirious at the time and that he would never want to leave her if he had a choice. Although Mrs. A. wants the physicians to do all they can to save her husband's life, she admits that she is concerned that she may be unable to provide the physical or emotional support he will need if he is ever able to return home.

Mr. A. did not prepare a written advance directive and never specifically discussed his wishes concerning life support or termination of treatment. However, both Mrs. A. and her father-in-law remember watching a television show about a man who had been kept alive on machines after an auto accident. Mr. A. commented at that time that he would "never want to be hooked up to anything like that."

Variations

- Mr. A. told a paramedic whom he had never seen before about his desire to die.
- Mr. A.'s burns are painful and have disfigured his face, but his hands and feet are not significantly damaged. After therapy, he will be able to meet his own self-care needs.

The Case of Mrs. B.

Mrs. B. is a 45-year-old woman who has been separated from her abusive, alcoholic husband for the last six years. She is financially comfortable and lives in her own home with her 27-year-old unmarried son.

Mrs. B. has a brain tumor that is causing an uncontrollable seizure disorder. She has been hospitalized for a week while evaluations were performed to determine whether surgery would be a viable treatment option. Early in the hospitalization, Mrs. B. told her son that she would want surgery if that was what her physicians recommended. However, that decision was not communicated specifically to the physicians, nor was it documented on her chart. In the last few days, Mrs. B.'s condition has deteriorated quickly, and she has been in and out of consciousness. She is often very confused and is inconsistent in her ability to communicate effectively.

Physicians have determined that surgery is an appropriate course of treatment and wish to schedule the operation as soon as possible. They have told Mrs. B.'s son that there is a chance that the surgery will not eliminate the seizures and that there is a slight chance that his mother would be worse after the surgery, yet they also have indicated that without the surgery her odds of surviving for more than a year are minimal.

The patient's husband, who has not been in contact with his family since the separation, recently arrived in town and demanded that he be informed of the details of his wife's situation. He is now stating that he has the right to choose the course of treatment for his "incompetent" wife and he is insisting that no surgery should be performed because his wife once told him she would not want to risk anything that might leave her as a "vegetable."

Mrs. B.'s son, who is openly hostile toward his father, is aware that his mother never changed her insurance policy and that his father is the beneficiary of that policy. He claims that money is the only motivating factor in his father's actions.

Variations

- Mrs. B.'s son is only 15 years old.
- The patient's husband was neither abusive nor an alcoholic. Their separation was amicable.
- There are no monetary issues involved.

The Case of Mrs. C.

Mrs. C. is an 81-year-old widow who has lived in a tiny walk-up apartment in the city since 1965. She has diabetes and is almost blind. Although she occasionally has lapses in memory, she is very comfortable in her familiar surroundings and has been able to care for herself adequately. Mrs. C.'s son, who had checked in on her daily, died suddenly three months ago. There are no other living relatives except a grandson who lives in Europe.

Mrs. C. fell down in her kitchen and broke her leg. She has spent the last several weeks in the hospital's physical rehabilitation unit.

Although Mrs. C. is in relatively good health and does not expect to die any time soon, she has written a living will, which states that she has led a "good and complete life" and that when the time comes she will be ready to "meet her Lord." She does not want to be resuscitated, nor does she want any artificial food or hydration. She does want to be given medication for pain and kept comfortable.

Mrs. C. has recovered sufficiently to be discharged from the hospital, and she is planning to return to her apartment. Staff on the rehabilitation unit do not feel that she is capable of living alone and are concerned for her safety. Social services staff have approached Mrs. C. about the possibility of going to a nursing home, but she is adamant that she does not want to use any of her savings for long-term care because she intends to leave all her money to her grandson. Mrs. C. has refused to allow staff to contact her grandson and has stated that she will call a cab to take her home if there is any more talk of nursing homes.

Variations

- Mrs. C.'s self-care skills are minimal. She is no longer able to cook and eats only cereal or cold sandwiches. She often forgets to lock her doors.

- Mrs. C. has no living relatives. She plans to leave all her money to an animal shelter.

- Mrs. C. allowed her grandson to be called. He says he neither wants nor needs her money and would prefer that she spend it on herself.

The Case of Ms. D.

Ms. D. is an intelligent, competent, articulate, educated 24-year-old woman who was born with severely deformed legs. She has been in a wheelchair since she was a child and has never been fitted for artificial legs because of the nature of her deformity. Ms. D. is unemployed. She lives at home with her parents, who not only support her financially but also are very attentive to her every need.

Ms. D. has requested that her legs be amputated. She hates how they look and wants them removed so that she does not have to deal with their "ugliness" on a daily basis. Ms. D. consulted a surgeon, who indicated that there was no medically indicated reason for the requested surgery. Thus, Ms. D.'s insurance company has refused to authorize payment for the surgery because it would be for cosmetic reasons only. Ms. D. does not have sufficient funds to pay for the operation privately.

Ms. D. consulted a psychiatrist, who sent a report to the surgeon stating that Ms. D.'s deformity causes her "mental anguish" and that she is at risk for additional psychological problems if the situation is not resolved. He stated that Ms. D.'s mental health would be greatly improved by surgery to amputate her legs. Ms. D. has asked her surgeon to reverse his decision and to determine that the surgery is medically indicated.

Variations

- Ms. D. has limited intellectual capacity. She was educated at home and has had minimal contact with persons other than her parents.

- Ms. D. is 16 years old. Her parents are strongly encouraging the surgery.

- Ms. D. has stated that she has no desire to go on living if her deformity cannot be corrected.

The Case of Baby E.

Baby E. is a two-day-old male infant born to an older couple who had been trying to have a baby for more than seven years. He was conceived through the use of fertility drugs. The mother's pregnancy was difficult, and she was prescribed bed rest for the last three months.

Labor was difficult and long. During the final moments of birth it was discovered that the umbilical cord was wrapped around the baby's neck. It was too late to perform a cesarean section, and the baby suffered fetal distress. Because of the lack of oxygen to his brain, he was born "blue" and was nonresponsive. Although the baby was resuscitated, he suffered severe brain damage and is unable to breathe on his own.

Baby E.'s mother is inconsolable and has been crying almost constantly since his birth. She has refused to see her child and does not want to name him. She keeps saying that the baby should be allowed to die so that she can put the "whole horrible disaster" behind her.

Baby E.'s father, although very upset, has asked for information as to whether his son could be used as an organ donor. He has requested that the child be kept alive on machines until a determination can be made. He has not discussed this possibility with his wife because he knows that it would only add to her distress. He feels certain, however, that it would help her in the long run if something positive could come out of their deep sorrow.

Variations

- Baby E. was born to young, healthy parents after an uneventful pregnancy.

- Baby E.'s mother has spent every waking moment at her infant's side. She knows he will die and wants to be holding him when it happens.

- Baby E. is a candidate to be a heart donor. Mr. E. has asked for help in talking about the possibility with his wife.

The Case of Mr. F.

Mr. F., age 88, is a charming, sociable, single, active man who lives in an exclusive retirement home in New England. He is a retired investment broker and has amassed a considerable fortune. He enjoys going to the theater, listening to classical music, reading all kinds of books, and taking daily walks around the grounds of the retirement home or to the local village. Although he has no living relatives, he has many friends and he dates several women with whom he frequently shares meals or stories of his past. Mr. F. takes an annual trip abroad with his men's group and regularly attends the local Catholic church.

Mr. F. had until now been in remarkably good health for his age. He had seen his doctor for regular checkups and for treatment of a minor respiratory problem. He had been eating and sleeping well.

Mr. F. prepared a very specific living will, in which he stated that he wants to have "everything known to medical science" done for him in the event of a medical emergency. He stated that he wants a full CODE, "all the machines available, food and water through tubes, and any medicines that might help cure" him.

Mr. F. has suffered a massive stroke. He has extensive brain damage, and there is no hope that he can ever be cured or that he can ever return to any type of life similar to that before the stroke.

Variations

- Mr. F. is a cranky, nasty, depressed recluse who rarely left his quarters and made no friends in the years he has lived in the retirement home.

- Mr. F.'s first stroke happened several weeks ago. He has had several small strokes since and has been resuscitated twice. His condition has been deteriorating on a daily basis.

- Mr. F.'s stroke was mild, but he is confused and is unable to talk.

The Case of Mrs. G.

Mrs. G. is a frail 72-year-old woman who recently lost her husband. They had no children, but she always considered her cats as her "babies."

Mrs. G. is in constant pain from crippling rheumatoid arthritis. She has neighbors who take her to buy groceries once a week and to the doctor's office periodically, but other than that, she rarely leaves her home. She reports that she is afraid to go out alone because the neighborhood is "going bad" and because vandals and robbers will attack her. She states that she is frequently scared, especially at night.

This woman has a long history of mental illness. She had several psychiatric admissions over the last 20 years, but she has not been hospitalized recently. She has a prescription for psychotropic medicines, which until recently she had taken regularly.

Last week Mrs. G., a professed atheist, attempted suicide. She was found when a neighbor smelled gas. She was saved; however, all but one of her six cats died. Mrs. G. is unaware of the death of her pets.

Mrs. G. is in the hospital and is very angry that she was not allowed to die. She states that she has "had enough" and that she has nothing to live for. She has refused any additional treatment in the hospital and is planning to leave against medical advice.

Variations

- Besides arthritis, Mrs. G. has heart disease and a tumor on her bladder. She is frequently incontinent.
- Mrs. G. is a devout Catholic who has been active in right-to-life issues in her parish.
- Mrs. G. has no history of mental illness.

The Case of Miss H.

Miss H. is a 20-year-old woman who comes from a strict, fundamentalist religious background. She rebelled against the teachings of the church and against her family and moved in with her fiancé.

Miss H. has contracted a serious, systemic infection following surgery for an ectopic pregnancy and has lapsed into a coma. She has no advance directive or living will. Her parents express shame over her actions and claim that she is being "punished for her sins." They maintain that if God believes that their daughter should be "forgiven," He will save her. In accordance with the teachings of their church, they believe that no medicines should be given to "artificially interfere with God's actions." They want their daughter discharged from the hospital so that they can take her to their home, where she will be "cared for, and prayed for, in proper surroundings."

The pastor from the H. family's church states that Miss H. never formally left the church and that she is therefore still a member. All members of the church denounce use of medications and believe in the healing power of prayer. He has a paper, signed by Miss H., stating her belief in this doctrine, which she signed when she first joined the congregation at age 16.

Miss H.'s fiancé insists that Miss H. wanted nothing whatsoever to do with her family or their church and that she would want all medications and treatments available.

Variations

- Miss H. is 30 years old.
- Miss H. was conflicted about her faith and demonstrated this by attending church services every now and then with her parents.
- Before lapsing into the coma, Miss H. told the hospital chaplain that she wanted to be cured.

The Case of Mr. I.

Three months ago Mr. I. experienced a cardiac arrest. He was resuscitated and placed on a ventilator, from which he cannot be weaned. He is unresponsive to stimuli but does have some minimal brain activity. He is being artificially fed and hydrated and has begun to develop contractures.

Mr. I. is a 79-year-old Methodist. He is a widower. He has a warm and loving relationship with his son and daughter-in-law, who visit him regularly. Mr. I.'s four young grandchildren also make weekly visits to "Pop-Pop." They like to read to him from their schoolbooks and tell him jokes.

Mr. I.'s medical insurance money has run out, and there are no funds to pay privately for him to remain in his present facility. The only nursing home that will accept him in transfer is more than 400 miles away. Placement in that facility would mean that his family would rarely be able to visit.

Mr. I.'s son, who has durable power of attorney for health care, believes that his father would rather die than be transferred to a place where he would be virtually alone. The son is reluctant to request that treatment be stopped, however, because of his deep affection for his dad.

Mr. I. never discussed his wishes concerning long-term care or life-support options.

Variations

- Mr. I. has no relatives. A lawyer has durable power of attorney.
- The nursing home that will accept Mr. I. is 50 miles away. The family will probably be able to visit at least once a month.
- Mr. I. is somewhat responsive. He smiles now and then and often appears to be watching things in his room. Occasionally, especially as the family is about to go home after a visit, Mr. I.'s son has seen tears in his father's eyes.

The Case of Child J.

Child J. is an eight-year-old boy who hit his head on a rock when he dove into a shallow creek. He was pulled, unconscious, from the water and was given cardiopulmonary resuscitation (CPR) at the scene. He appears to have suffered no brain damage, but he remains sedated; a full battery of tests has not yet been administered.

It is clear, however, that this child has suffered a broken neck and a severed spinal cord. He has lost all feeling and movement in both his arms and his legs. He is incontinent. There is no hope that he will ever regain any purposeful movement in his limbs. It is expected that he will be dependent on others for all of his personal-care needs for the rest of his life.

Child J. is the oldest of five siblings. His father is a maintenance worker, and his pregnant mother earns money by cleaning houses. Neither parent finished high school, and it appears that they are both limited intellectually. The family has no religious affiliation. His parents are very confused about what has happened to their son. In the days immediately following the accident, they frequently asked how much longer it was going to take for the doctors to "fix" him.

After numerous conferences with the health care staff and social workers, the child's parents announced one afternoon that a friend had told them that they should not try to take care of their son at home and that they should put the boy in an institution for the disabled. They told a staff nurse that they had decided to do just that, and asked her to "take care of things." They then walked out of the hospital and have not returned. Attempts to reach the family by phone have been unsuccessful. Child J. has awakened several times and has tearfully asked for his parents.

Variations

- Besides being quadriplegic, Child J. suffered extensive brain damage as a result of his accident.
- Child J. is an only child. His parents are well-to-do professionals. They are very aware of the implications for their son's future and do not want him in their home.
- Child J.'s parents do not agree. His father wants him to be put in an institution; his mother does not.

The Case of Mr. K.

Mr. K. is a 48-year-old alcoholic who has no desire to stop drinking. Although Mr. K. himself has not attended church for many years, he is married to a very religious woman, who is extremely angry at him for his alcohol abuse and for all the things she believes he has done to make her life constantly miserable. Mr. K. would be happy to divorce and has offered on numerous occasions to do so, but his wife refuses because divorce is against her religious beliefs. Mr. and Mrs. K. have two grown sons, both of whom are heavy drinkers. All the men in the family report that they drink only to get away from the constant religious preaching and hatred expressed by their wife or mother.

Mr. K.'s alcoholism has caused cirrhosis of the liver. He has been informed that he needs a liver transplant to survive. The patient wants the transplant. His wife, however, is against the surgery because she feels it is a waste of money and because she is angry that she will have to care for him when he comes home. Mr. K.'s physicians are also reluctant to use scarce resources to provide a new liver for a patient who has no intention of altering his lifestyle.

Variations

- Mr. K. and his sons are not drinkers. His disease is the result of hepatitis. Mrs. K. is angry because of an unhappy marriage.

- Mr. K. has agreed to try to stop drinking if he is given a new liver.

- Mr. K. is wealthy. He is willing to pay privately for any services and care he may need.

The Case of Mrs. L.

Mrs. L. is a 79-year-old widow who lives alone in a small house in a relatively nice city neighborhood. She has seven adult children, none of whom get along very well with each other. They rarely visit their mother but do phone her every now and then.

Mrs. L. comes to the emergency department (ED) of City Hospital every few weeks (more often during the winter) complaining of various aches, pains, and ailments. Whenever Mrs. L. visits the ED, she is given a thorough evaluation and a complete battery of appropriate tests. Some of her complaints are legitimate (she has hypertension and diabetes); however, on investigation and evaluation, it is often learned that there is no physiological reason for Mrs. L.'s problems.

Mrs. L. is a sweet little old lady who has developed a pleasant rapport with the hospital staff. She is always very thankful for the care she receives and frequently arrives for her visits with a batch of homemade cookies. Whenever there is a trauma or when the ED is very busy, Mrs. L. sits quietly in the corner until the staff is no longer needed elsewhere. Although the staff is truly fond of Mrs. L. and wants to be certain that all of her medical needs are taken care of, they feel that her visits to the ED for nonemergency complaints happen much too frequently and that the funds expended on her are excessive.

Variations

- Mrs. L. is neither sweet nor pleasant. She is always very demanding of the ED staff and expects to be treated immediately.
- Mrs. L. is often brought to the ED by one of her children, who stays long enough to see that she is registered, then leaves, only to return several hours later to drive her home.
- Mrs. L.'s visits to the ED occur approximately three or four times a year.

The Case of Miss M.

Miss M. is a 59-year-old single woman who has lived all her life with her younger sister, who is schizophrenic. There are no other living relatives; however, for the last 15 years, the sisters have shared their home with a friend who helps pay the bills and provides some personal care for both women. They all attend mass regularly at the local Catholic church.

Miss M. has a heart condition. She was hospitalized recently after a heart attack, which followed a heated disagreement with her sister. Since the incident, Miss M. has been confused and disoriented. Miss M. apparently was without oxygen to her brain for a short time before the paramedics were able to resuscitate her. Her mental status, however, is improving every day, and otherwise she appears to be in good health.

A few months ago, Miss M. wrote a living will and gave it to her physician. In the document, she requested that no extraordinary measures be used to save her life in the event of a terminal illness. She indicated that she did not want cardiopulmonary resuscitation (CPR) to be used if her heart should stop. As a result of this living will, Miss M.'s physician has written a do-not-resuscitate (DNR) order. This was explained to Miss M.'s sister in the presence of their live-in friend.

Miss M.'s friend subsequently asked to meet with the physician and explained that the document had been written in a moment of anger after the sisters had had one of their numerous arguments. She reported that Miss M. had verbally revoked the living will, stating that she knew that her sister needed her.

Miss M.'s friend has asked the physician to revoke the DNR order and to make every effort to preserve Miss M.'s life. Miss M.'s sister has no opinion in the matter.

Variations

- Miss M.'s condition is getting worse every day. She is not making the progress that her physicians had first expected.
- Even though Miss M. is confused and has short-term memory loss, she has reminded her physician that she has a living will.
- Miss M.'s sister is extremely distraught at the idea that her sister may die.

The Case of Mrs. N.

Mrs. N. is a 61-year-old married woman who has always been extremely active and independent. She has maintained a professional career while raising two children and writing several books. Mrs. N. has invested wisely and now has a large personal fortune. She serves on the board of directors of several charitable organizations and takes piano lessons in her spare time.

Mrs. N. was recently admitted to the hospital for evaluation of abdominal pain and dysfunctional uterine bleeding. She was diagnosed with a malignant mass, which her physician believes should be surgically removed immediately.

Mrs. N., however, is scheduled to leave on a solo "trip of a lifetime"—a four-week trip to ancient archeological sites in Upper Egypt—which she is determined to take prior to any surgery. She believes that if she does not take the trip now she may never be able to take it. She is fully aware that the mass will continue to grow while she is away and that such a lengthy delay may have a serious detrimental effect on the final outcome. She says she does not care what happens and that she is willing to take the risk. Mrs. N. believes that the pain can be controlled with medication and states that if she gets into "serious trouble," she will cut the trip short and come home.

Mrs. N.'s husband, who has always been fully supportive of his wife's activities, is totally against the trip. He believes that his wife is so frightened by the diagnosis of this serious illness that she is not analyzing the situation rationally. He states that this behavior is totally out of character for his wife, who has always been very logical and sensible in her personal decisions. Mr. N. wants the physician and the hospital to support him in his claim that his wife is not competent to make health care decisions. He plans to apply for legal guardianship so that he can force his wife to have the surgery immediately.

Variations

- Mrs. N.'s mass is nonmalignant.
- Mrs. N.'s husband has not been supportive. He has always been jealous of his wife's accomplishments and feels that this particular trip is a waste of time and money.
- Mrs. N.'s trip is going to take her to very remote locations. Communication and travel in or out of the region are extremely difficult.

The Case of Baby O.

Baby O. is a 9-week-old female infant who has been brought to the emergency department (ED) by ambulance three times since birth because of episodes of "cessation of breathing." Her 35-year-old single mother reports that she has been able to revive the infant quickly but that she calls the paramedics as a precaution. Baby O. had a sister who died of sudden infant death syndrome when she was 10 months old. Baby O. had been on an apnea monitor since birth.

Baby O.'s mother is always very calm during her visits to the ED with her infant. She clearly articulates every aspect of the episode, giving details of time, duration, preceding events, and the general health status of her daughter. She never shows any overt signs of distress or emotion.

After the most recent episode, a neighbor of Baby O.'s called the hospital and reported that she was with the family immediately before the incident and that the infant's mother was acting very strangely. The neighbor suspects that the mother did something to the child to make her stop breathing. She suspects child abuse but has nothing specific to go on. The neighbor would not leave her name.

Variations

- When Baby O.'s mother arrives at the ED, she is always very upset and appears frantic that she may lose this child too.

- Baby O. is 19 months old. She has numerous new and healing bruises on her body, which her mother says were the result of falls while playing.

- Baby O.'s mother has a history of being hospitalized for a severe manic-depressive condition.

The Case of Mr. P.

Mr. P., an 85-year-old widower with no children, has been in a persistent vegetative state for the last four months following a series of strokes. Although he can breathe on his own, he cannot communicate, has no awareness of his surroundings, and is unresponsive to sound, light, and touch. His closest living relatives are his 79-year-old twin siblings, a brother and a sister. They are all communicants at an Episcopal church.

Before the last admission, Mr. P.'s physician suggested that he prepare a living will, but Mr. P. refused to do so. His specific wishes concerning end-of-life treatment are unknown. Mr. P. is being given artificial food and hydration, but he has lost a great deal of weight and now weighs only 103 pounds.

Mr. P.'s brother wants to stop the artificial food and hydration so that his brother can die. He feels that keeping him alive is not doing him any good and that it is cruel to allow things to continue as they are. Mr. P.'s sister, on the other hand, is equally convinced that all treatment should continue. She feels that it would be murder to stop treatment and believes that if her brother were ready to die, he would do so, with or without the artificial food and hydration.

Variations

- Mr. P.'s siblings are not twins. His sister is 79. His brother is 76.
- Mr. P. is also on a ventilator. Attempts to wean him off the ventilator have been unsuccessful.
- Mr. P. talked about a living will with his physician and stated that he thought he should write one because he wanted to die "without a fuss."

The Case of Mrs. Q.

Mrs. Q., a 29-year old, was involved in an automobile accident five weeks ago. Since the accident, she has been comatose and on a ventilator. It is known that Mrs. Q. suffered a very severe brain injury in the accident, but there were no other injuries. Mrs. Q.'s husband and their 16-month-old daughter were both killed in the accident. Mrs. Q., who comes from a very devout Baptist family, has two living relatives—her brother and her father.

Mrs. Q., a nurse by profession, has had several conversations over the last few years with family members concerning serious illness, life support, and termination-of-treatment issues as they related to her patients. Although Mrs. Q. never wrote anything down concerning her own personal wishes, she made it very clear that she did not believe in using "heroic measures" when there was little or no hope of recovery.

Mrs. Q.'s physicians have indicated that her prognosis is grave. They have discussed the possibility of removing Mrs. Q. from the ventilator.

Mrs. Q.'s father and brother believe that Mrs. Q. would not want to remain hooked up to the ventilator and that the best thing would probably be for her to die to join her family in heaven. Both, however, are so devastated by the loss of the other members of their family that they can not face the thought of another death. They have asked the hospital staff for help in making the right choice.

Variations

- Mrs. Q.'s husband and daughter were not killed in the accident.

- Mrs. Q. is a clerical worker. She never discussed end-of-life issues with anyone.

- Mrs. Q. is seven-and-a-half-months pregnant. The fetus was unharmed.

The Case of Ms. R.

Ms. R. is a divorced, 34-year-old mother of two. Her children, ages two and five, are cared for during the day by a nanny, while their mother works as a fashion designer. Ms. R.'s parents are alive, but both are elderly and physically unwell. They live in a distant city and have had contact with their daughter only on holidays for the last several years. Ms. R. is an only child. Her ex-husband has not been involved with his children since their divorce. He wants nothing to do with the family, and his present whereabouts are unknown.

Ms. R. has breast cancer. It was not discovered early, and it has spread to her bones and one lung. Ms. R. has participated in an aggressive series of treatments, including surgery, two courses of chemotherapy, and radiation therapy. She is now about to begin another course of chemotherapy, which she is certain will cure her.

Ms. R.'s physician is very upbeat and optimistic. She feels that it is important to keep a positive attitude and that a happy mental outlook creates the perfect climate for maximum therapeutic benefit.

The nursing staff who are working with Ms. R. feel that the physician is not being honest with this patient. They are convinced that the optimistic attitude of the physician is giving the patient false hopes. They believe that they cannot work effectively with Ms. R. because she does not know how sick she really is. Several staff members have attempted to discuss their concerns with the physician, but she has made it very clear that she is in charge and that they are not to interfere.

Ms. R. has done nothing to prepare for the possibility of her death. She has written no advance directive, has appointed no one to assume power of attorney, and—of great concern to the staff—she has made no provisions for the care of her children.

Variations

- Ms. R. has never been married and has no children.
- Ms. R. has mentioned to one of the nurses that she does not believe she is being told the truth about her disease.
- Ms. R.'s cancer has spread to her brain. She is often very confused and agitated.

The Case of Mr. S.

Mr. S. is a 44-year-old, handsome, robust, athletic widower who is engaged to be married to a woman 10 years his junior. His fiancée, a Catholic, is very anxious to be married and to start a large family.

Mr. S., however, is now sterile as a result of having mumps as an adult. His sterility was discovered when he and his previous wife were unable to conceive.

Mr. S.'s present physician is aware of his sterility and has questioned whether the information had been shared with Mr. S.'s fiancée. Mr. S. has told his physician that he will not share the information for fear that his fiancée will call off the wedding. He has threatened to sue the physician for breach of confidentiality if he divulges the information.

Variations

- Mr. S.'s fiancée is 40. She wants a family very much but is aware that her age may prevent her from conceiving.

- Mr. S.'s sterility is due to a vasectomy during his previous marriage.

- Mr. S. and his fiancée go to the same family physician.

The Case of Miss T.

Miss T. is a 15-year-old girl who lives at home with her parents. She has one older brother, who is an *A* student, a member of the football team, and a leader in student government. He is in his third year of college, in a premed program.

Miss T.'s father, an accountant, is quiet and soft-spoken. He spends most of his free time by himself either reading in his study or painting watercolors. His wife, on the other hand, is lively and outspoken. She is involved in numerous neighborhood organizations and enjoys lunching with her friends or volunteering at the local playhouse.

Mrs. T. is very proud of her son and is happy to discuss his successes with anyone who will listen. She does not feel the same sense of pride, however, for her daughter. She feels that Miss T. does not try hard enough in school and that she is too introverted. She often calls her daughter a "wallflower." Mother and daughter have frequent, heated arguments.

For the last two years, Miss T. has been steadily losing weight. She is 5 feet 4 inches tall and weighs 92 pounds. Her mother is constantly encouraging her to eat more, but Miss T. claims that she is not hungry and that her weight is fine. Mrs. T. has met with their family physician and is insisting that her daughter be hospitalized and force-fed. Mrs. T. does not believe in psychological therapy and refuses to participate in any family or individual counseling sessions.

Variations

- Miss T. is an only child. Her parents are both quiet and reserved. There are no family fights. Miss T.'s mother is not displeased with anything about her daughter except her weight.
- Miss T. is underweight but only by about 15 pounds. Her mother still feels very strongly that her daughter is too thin.
- Miss T.'s mother is 5 feet 3 inches tall and weighs 234 pounds.

The Case of Mr. U.

Mr. U. is a 65-year-old patient who has amyotrophic lateral sclerosis (ALS), also known as Lou Gehrig's disease. He is alert, oriented, and mentally competent.

When this disease was first diagnosed, Mr. U. did a lot of research and familiarized himself with his prognosis and the likely course that the disease would take. He subsequently wrote a document concerning how he wanted the end of his life to be handled. The document clearly states that when the time comes to die, he wants no extraordinary means to maintain life, no artificial food or hydration, and no CODEs. The document does state that he wants to be heavily medicated so that he can feel no pain.

Mr. U. has reached the point at which he can no longer do anything for himself. He has indicated that he is ready to die, and he has stated that he no longer wants to be fed. He is in a home care hospice program.

Mr. U.'s wife, who obviously loves her husband dearly, is confused as to what can and should be done now. She knows what her husband's wishes are, and she wants to abide by them, yet she is afraid that he will suffer if he is not fed or given water. She is also fearful that such an action might be illegal.

Variations

- Besides the ALS, Mr. U. also had a stroke, which left him mentally disoriented.

- Mr. U. did not write anything about his end-of-life wishes, but he did tell them to his wife and their minister.

- Mr. U. is in a nursing home.

The Case of Mrs. V.

Mrs. V., age 76, is married and the mother of six children. She lives with her husband (who has Alzheimer's disease) and one unmarried adult daughter. The rest of the children live in various parts of the country, but they are in frequent contact with their parents and provide financial support whenever they can.

Mrs. V. has a benign abdominal tumor, which has been growing for several years. She has refused surgery because of fear and because she was reluctant to be away from her husband. The tumor is now so large that she is having trouble breathing and eating. She is in constant pain and, as a result, her daughter has been doing all the housework besides providing personal care for both parents.

Mrs. V. was taken to the hospital by ambulance after a recent episode of severe pain and vomiting. Surgery has again been recommended, and Mrs. V. has again refused. Mrs. V.'s daughter is furious. She states that unless her mother has this surgery, she will move out of the house and that both parents will have to fend for themselves.

Variations

- Mrs. V.'s tumor was only recently diagnosed. It is malignant.
- Mrs. V.'s mother died during surgery 32 years ago. Mrs. V. is convinced that if she has this surgery, she too will die on the operating table.
- Mr. and Mrs. V. are well off financially. Mrs. V. says that if her daughter moves out, she will hire someone to move in and provide all the necessary services.

The Case of Mr. W.

Mr. W. is a 49-year-old homosexual who has lived with his current partner for 21 years. Mr. W. is Catholic by birth, but for the last several years he has been a member of a nondenominational congregation, which has many members from the local gay community.

Mr. W. has AIDS. He has Kaposi's sarcoma and neurological deficits and recently has begun to have seizures. Mr. W. is confused and disoriented. He is near death.

Before the final stages of his illness, Mr. W. typed and signed an advance directive giving his partner durable power of attorney for health care. In addition to the original document, which he gave to his partner, Mr. W. gave a second copy to his minister. However, the document was only recently given to Mr. W.'s physician.

Mr. W. has only a few weeks, at best, to live. His partner wants to take him to their own home for his last days. However, Mr. W.'s parents (who totally deny his homosexuality) claim that the signature on the advance directive document was forged, and they have engaged an attorney to force the hospital to discharge their son into their care.

Variations

- Mr. W. has lived with his current partner for only eight months.
- Mr. W. did not write an advance directive. Although his mental capacity is diminished, he has stated several times that he wants to go home to his own house. His parents claim he doesn't know what he is saying.
- Mr. W.'s parents are very loving and accepted his homosexuality years ago. They are fond of Mr. W.'s partner, but they still want to take their son home to die. They do not want the partner to come with them.

The Case of Ms. X.

Ms. X. is a woman who appears to be in her mid- to late 20s. She was brought to the trauma unit of Community Hospital three weeks ago after being found unconscious along the side of the highway. She was alone at the time she was found, and there were no witnesses who could provide information as to what had happened to her. It is believed that Ms. X. was probably the victim of a hit-and-run accident.

Ms. X. was well dressed when she was found and was wearing an expensive watch. She had no identification on her, and all attempts to learn her identity have been unsuccessful.

Ms. X. has remained unconscious since her admission. She has had surgery to correct internal injuries and broken bones. Her progress has been minimal, and her prognosis is grave.

Ms. X. suffered one episode of cardiopulmonary arrest, from which she was resuscitated. Additional arrests are possible, and Ms. X.'s physicians are questioning whether she should be considered a "no CODE."

Variations

- Ms. X. is elderly.

- Ms. X. appears to be a street person. She was very dirty and was dressed in torn and ragged clothes when found. Ms. X. also had a very high blood alcohol level.

- Ms. X. appears to have been beaten. Police theorize that she may have been dropped along the side of the highway.

The Case of Mr. Y.

Two months ago Mr. Y., a wealthy 70-year-old businessman, went to Reno, Nevada; divorced his wife of many years; and married a woman half his age, whom he had known for only a few weeks. Mr. Y.'s two grown children, who are both older than the new Mrs. Y., are furious with their father and believe that he was "taken" for his money.

Mr. Y. has a slow-growing, cancerous growth in his lung. His physician has explained all the possible treatment options to him, but Mr. Y. cannot decide what he wants to do about it. On one day he may say that he wants to have surgery, and on the next he may say he wants only chemotherapy. This indecision has been going on for three weeks.

Mr. Y.'s physician requested a psychiatric evaluation, which demonstrated that Mr. Y. has an impaired level of competence. Mrs. Y. has decided that she is going to apply for guardianship of her husband so that she can make medical decisions for him.

Mr. Y.'s children are contending that if their father is incompetent now, he was incompetent two months ago, when he was married, and that one of them should be making the medical decisions for their father.

Variations

- Mr. Y. is a retired bookkeeper. He has little money in the bank.
- Mr. Y.'s cancer is growing very rapidly.
- The psychiatric evaluation showed that Mr. Y. is fully competent.

The Case of Baby Z.

Baby Z., an only child, is six months old. She was born with a defective heart and had a heart transplant within the first two months of life. In addition to her heart problems, Baby Z. is also blind, deaf, and probably mentally retarded.

Baby Z.'s parents are very loving, concerned, and caring. As Catholics, they have a strong Christian faith and believe that they have been given this baby as a special gift to care for and cherish. They are firm in their belief that they must do everything in their power to protect and preserve her life.

Baby Z.'s parents, who are financially secure, are fully prepared to take her home and care for her for as long as she is able to live. They see her retardation and other disabilities as a challenge, not as an obstacle.

Baby Z.'s transplanted heart is failing. Her parents want her to have a second heart transplant.

Variations

- Baby Z. does not have any medical problems other than her heart condition.
- Baby Z.'s parents have little money. They would need a great deal of financial support in order to provide all the care that their child would need.
- Baby Z.'s parents have had two other children. Both were born with the same heart condition that this child has, and both died within weeks of birth. Neither of those babies was given a new heart.

Bibliography and Resources

In addition to the references and suggested readings cited at the end of the chapters, the following videos, books, and journal articles are offered as supplementary sources of information on biomedical ethics topics. Also included are the names and addresses of some of the centers for ethics education, information, and conferences as well as the names and addresses of many of the periodicals that contain biomedical ethics articles.

This list represents only a small portion of the vast amount of information available in the field. As such, it is intended to provide the reader with possible sources of basic information and a starting point for developing a library of biomedical ethics references.

Books and General References on Biomedical Ethics

Abrams, N., and Buckner, M. D. *Medical Ethics: A Clinical Textbook and Reference for Health Care Professionals.* Cambridge, MA: MIT Press, 1983.

American Hospital Association Special Committee on Biomedical Ethics. *Values in Conflict: Resolving Ethical Issues in Hospital Care.* Chicago: American Hospital Association, 1985.

American Hospital Association Technical Panel on Biomedical Ethics. *Values in Conflict: Resolving Ethical Issues in Health Care.* 2nd ed. Chicago: American Hospital Association, 1994.

Arras, J., and Rhoden, N. K. *Ethical Issues in Modern Medicine.* 3rd ed. Mountain View, CA: Mayfield, 1989.

Ashley, B. M., and O'Rourke, K. *Healthcare Ethics—A Theological Analysis.* St. Louis: Catholic Health Association of the United States, 1989.

Beauchamp, T. L., and Childress, J. F. *Principles of Biomedical Ethics.* 3rd ed. New York City: Oxford University Press, 1989.

Beauchamp, T. L., and Perlin, S. *Ethical Issues in Death and Dying.* Englewood Cliffs, NJ: Prentice Hall, 1977.

Beauchamp, T. L., and Walters, L., editors. *Contemporary Issues in Bioethics.* 3rd ed. Belmont, CA: Wadsworth Publishing Co., 1989.

Brock, D. H., and Ratzan, R. M., editors. *Literature and Bioethics.* Baltimore: Johns Hopkins University Press, 1988.

Doudera, A. E., and Peters, J. D., editors. *Legal and Ethical Aspects of Treating Critically and Terminally Ill Patients.* Ann Arbor, MI: Association of University Programs in Health Administration Press, 1982.

Friedman, E., editor. *Choices and Conflict: Explorations in Health Care Ethics.* Chicago: American Hospital Publishing, 1992.

Friedman, E., editor. *Making Choices: Ethics Issues for Health Care Professionals.* Chicago: American Hospital Publishing, 1986.

Jonsen, A., Seigler, M., and Winslade, W. J. *Clinical Ethics.* New York City: Macmillan, 1982.

Levine, C., editor. *Taking Sides: Clashing Views on Controversial Bioethical Issues.* 3rd ed. Guilford, CT: Dushkin Publishing Group, 1989.

Mappes, T. A., and Zembaty, J. S. *Biomedical Ethics.* 3rd ed. New York City: McGraw-Hill, 1991.

O'Rourke, K. D., and Brouder, D. *Medical Ethics: Common Ground for Understanding.* St. Louis: Catholic Health Association of the United States, 1986.

President's Commission for the Study of Ethical Problems in Medicine and Biomedical and Behavioral Research. *Compensating for Research Injuries.* 2 vols. Washington, DC: U.S. Government Printing Office, 1982.

President's Commission for the Study of Ethical Problems in Medicine and Biomedical and Behavioral Research. *Deciding to Forgo Life-Sustaining Treatment.* Washington, DC: U.S. Government Printing Office, 1983.

President's Commission for the Study of Ethical Problems in Medicine and Biomedical and Behavioral Research. *Defining Death.* Washington, DC: U.S. Government Printing Office, 1981.

President's Commission for the Study of Ethical Problems in Medicine and Biomedical and Behavioral Research. *Implementing Human Research Regulations.* Washington, DC: U.S. Government Printing Office, 1983.

President's Commission for the Study of Ethical Problems in Medicine and Biomedical and Behavioral Research. *Making Health Care Decisions.* 3 vols. Washington, DC: U.S. Government Printing Office, 1982–83.

President's Commission for the Study of Ethical Problems in Medicine and Biomedical and Behavioral Research. *Protecting Human Subjects.* Washington, DC: U.S. Government Printing Office, 1981.

President's Commission for the Study of Ethical Problems in Medicine and Biomedical and Behavioral Research. *Screening and Counseling for Genetic Conditions.* Washington, DC: U.S. Government Printing Office, 1983.

President's Commission for the Study of Ethical Problems in Medicine and Biomedical and Behavioral Research. *Securing Access to Health Care.* 3 vols. Washington, DC: U.S. Government Printing Office, 1983.

President's Commission for the Study of Ethical Problems in Medicine and Biomedical and Behavioral Research. *Splicing Life.* Washington, DC: U.S. Government Printing Office, 1982.

President's Commission for the Study of Ethical Problems in Medicine and Biomedical and Behavioral Research. *Summing Up.* Washington, DC: U.S. Government Printing Office, 1983.

President's Commission for the Study of Ethical Problems in Medicine and Biomedical and Behavioral Research. *Whistleblowing in Biomedical Research.* Washington, DC: U.S. Government Printing Office, 1981.

Ramsey, P. *Ethics at the Edges of Life.* New Haven, CT: Yale University Press, 1978.

Reich, W. T., editor. *Encyclopedia of Bioethics.* 4 vols. New York City: Free Press, 1978.

Reiser, S., Dyck, A., and Curran, W. *Ethics in Medicine: Historical Perspectives and Contemporary Concerns.* Cambridge, MA: MIT Press, 1977.

Veatch, R. *A Theory of Medical Ethics.* New York City: Basic Books, 1981.

Periodicals

American Journal of Law and Medicine
American Society of Law and Medicine
765 Commonwealth Ave.
Boston, MA 02215

Cambridge Quarterly of Healthcare Ethics
Cambridge University Press
40 W. 20th St.
New York, NY 10011-4211

Ethical Currents
Center for Bioethics, St. Joseph Health System and the California Association of Catholic Hospitals
1121 L St., Suite 409
Sacramento, CA 95814

Ethics in Nursing
Williams & Wilkins
P.O. Box 23291
Baltimore, MD 21203-9990

Frontlines
Center for Applied Biomedical Ethics
at Rose Medical Center
4567 E. Ninth Ave.
Denver, CO 80220

Hastings Center Report
The Hastings Center
255 Elm Rd.
Briarcliff Manor, NY 10510

Health Progress
Catholic Health Association
4455 Woodson Rd.
St. Louis, MO 63134-0889

HEC Forum
Kluwer
P.O. Box 358
Accord Station
Hingham, MA 02018-0358

Hospital Ethics
American Hospital Association
One N. Franklin
Chicago, IL 60606

Journal of Clinical Ethics
University Publishing Group
107 E. Church St.
Frederick, MD 21701

Journal of Law, Medicine and Philosophy
Society for Health and Human Values
University of Chicago Press
5801 S. Ellis Ave.
Chicago, IL 60637

Kennedy Institute of Ethics Journal
Johns Hopkins University Press
701 W. 40th St., Suite 275
Baltimore, MD 21211-2190

Law, Medicine, and Health Care
American Society of Law and Medicine
765 Commonwealth Ave.
Boston, MA 02215

Medical Ethics Advisor
American Health Consultants, Inc.
3525 Piedmont Rd. N.E.
Bldg. 6, Suite 400
Atlanta, GA 30305

Centers for Biomedical Ethics Education, Information and/or Conferences

American Bar Association
Commission on Legal Problems
of the Elderly
1800 M Street N.W., South Lobby
Washington, DC 20036

American Hospital Association
Special Membership Services, 30th Floor
or
Resource Center
One N. Franklin
Chicago, IL 60606

American Medical Association
515 N. State St.
Chicago, IL 60610

American Nurses Association
600 Maryland Ave. S.W.
Suite 100 W
Washington, DC 20024-2571

American Society of Law and Medicine
765 Commonwealth Ave.
Boston, MA 02215

Canadian Bioethics Society
Medical Affairs
Hamilton Civic Hospitals
237 Barton St. East
Hamilton, Ontario, Canada L8L 2X2

Center For Clinical Ethics
Lutheran General Hospital
8 South
1775 Dempster St.
Park Ridge, IL 60068

Center for Health Care Ethics
St. Louis University Medical Center
1402 S. Grand Blvd.
St. Louis, MO 63104

Concern for Dying/Society for the Right to Die
250 W. 57th St.
New York, NY 10107

Deaconess Health System
Religion and Health Department
Deaconess Medical Center–Central Campus
6150 Oakland Ave.
St. Louis, MO 63139

Ethics Center
Loma Linda University
Loma Linda, CA 92350

Hastings Center
255 Elm Rd.
Briarcliff Manor, NJ 10510

International Bioethics Institute
1722 Mar West
Tiburon, CA 94920-1932

Kennedy Institute of Ethics
Georgetown University
Washington, DC 20057

Midwest Bioethics Center
410 Archibald Rd., Suite 200
Kansas City, MO 64111

The Park Ridge Center
211 E. Ontario St., Suite 800
Chicago, IL 60611

The Poynter Center for the Study of Ethics
410 N. Park Ave.
Bloomington, IN 46405

Topic-Specific Information

Allocation of Resources

Aaron, H. J., and Schwartz, W. B. *The Painful Prescription: Rationing Hospital Care.* Washington, DC: Brookings Institute, 1984.

Beresford, E. B. Uncertainty and the shaping of medical decisions. *Hastings Center Report* 21(4):6–11, July–Aug. 1991.

Blendon, R. J., Edwards, J. N., and Hyams, A. L. Making critical choices. *JAMA* 267(18):2509–20, May 13, 1992.

Carrns, A., editor. Should elderly patients be given costly high-tech care? *Medical Ethics Advisor* 9(12):149–60, Dec. 1993.

Englehardt, H. T., Jr., and Rie, M. A. Intensive care units, scarce resources, and conflicting principles of justice. *JAMA* 255(9):1159–64, Mar. 7, 1986.

Fuchs, V. *The Health Economy.* Cambridge, MA: Harvard University Press, 1986.

Scitovsky, A. A., and Capron, A. M. Medical care at the end of life: the interaction of economics and ethics. *Annual Review of Public Health* 7:59–75, 1986.

Veatch, R. M. DRGs and the ethical allocation of resources. *Hastings Center Report* 16(3):32–40, June 1986.

Competency

Carms, A., editor. Incompetent patients without guardians: a special dilemma. *Medical Ethics Advisor* 8(12):133–44, Dec. 1992.

Rushton, C. H., and Hogue, E. E. The role of families as surrogate decision makers after Cruzan v. Director, Missouri Department of Health. *Journal of Contemporary Health Law and Policy* 7):219–338, Spring 1991.

Waldron, E. E. Decision making and the incompetent patient: a tale of two committees. *HEC Forum* 3(1):3–18, 1991.

Do Not Resuscitate (DNR)

American Medical Association, Council on Ethical and Judicial Affairs. Guidelines for the appropriate use of do-not-resuscitate orders. *JAMA* 265(14):1868–971, Apr. 10, 1991.

Hackler, J. C., and Hiller, C. Family consent to orders not to resuscitate. *JAMA* 264(10):1281–83, Sept. 12, 1990.

Lee, M. A., and Cassell, C. The ethical and legal framework for the decision not to resuscitate. *Western Journal of Medicine* 140(1):117–22, Jan. 1984.

Lipton, H. Do-not-resuscitate orders in a community hospital. *JAMA* 256(9):1164–69, Sept. 5, 1986.

Moreno, J. Who's to choose? *Hastings Center Report* 23(1):5–11, Jan.–Feb. 1993.

Spinsanti, S. Obtaining consent from the family: a horizon in clinical ethics. *Journal of Clinical Ethics* 3(3):188–92, Fall 1992.

Walker, R. M. DNR in the OR. *JAMA* 266(17):2407–11, Nov. 6, 1991.

Ethics Education

Barlotta, F. M., and Scheirton, L. S. The role of the hospital ethics committee in educating members of the medical staff. *HEC Forum* 1(3):151–58, 1989.

Carson, R. A., and Higgs, R. Case method. *Journal of Medical Ethics* 12(1):36–39, Mar. 1986.

Christensen, K. T. Self-education for hospital ethics committees. *HEC Forum* 1(6):333–39, 1989.

Clouser, K. D. *Teaching Bioethics: Strategies, Problems and Resources.* Hastings-on-Hudson, NY: Hastings Center, 1980.

Francoeur, R. T. A structured approach to teaching decision-making skills in biomedical ethics. *Journal of Bioethics* 5(2):145–54, Fall–Winter 1984.

Howe, K. R., Holmes, M., and Elstein, A. S. Teaching clinical decision making. *Journal of Medicine and Philosophy* 9(2):215–28, May 1984.

Levine, C., editor. *Cases in Bioethics.* New York City: St. Martin's Press, 1989.

Miles, S. H., Lane, L. W., Bickel, J., Walker, R. M., and Cassel, C. K. Ethics education: coming of age. *Academic Medicine* 64(12):705–14, Dec. 1989.

Odom, J. G. The status of ethics instruction in the health education curriculum. *Health Education* 19(4):9–12, Aug.–Sept. 1988.

Pellegrino, E. D. Teaching medical ethics: some persistent questions and some responses. *Academic Medicine* 64(12):701–3, Dec. 1989.

Pence, G. E. *Classic Cases in Medical Ethics: Accounts of the Cases That Have Shaped Medical Ethics, with Philosophical, Legal, and Historical Backgrounds.* New York City: McGraw-Hill, 1990.

Siegler, M., Rezler, A. G., and Cornell, K. J. Using simulated case studies to evaluate a clinical ethics course for junior students. *Journal of Medical Education* 57(5):380–85, May 1982.

Tymuchuk, A. J. Strategies for resolving value dilemmas. *American Behavioral Scientist* 26(2):159–75, Nov.–Dec. 1982.

Veatch, R. M. *Case Studies in Medical Ethics.* Cambridge, MA: Harvard University Press, 1977.

Veatch, R. M. Medical ethics education. In: W. T. Reich, editor. *Encyclopedia of Bioethics.* Vol. 1. New York City: Free Press, 1978, pp. 870–75.

Waithe, M. E., Duckett, L., Schmitz, K., Crisham, P., and Ryden, M. B. Developing case situations for ethics education in nursing. *Journal of Nursing Education* 28(4):175–80, Apr. 1989.

White, G., and Davis, A. Teaching ethics using games. *Journal of Advanced Nursing* 12(5):621–24, Sept. 1987.

Ethics Committees

Bowen, H. *Bioethics Committees.* Rockville, MD: Aspen Systems Corp., 1986.

Cranford, R. E., and Doudera, A. E., editors. *Institutional Ethics Committees and Health Care Decision Making.* Ann Arbor, MI: Health Administration Press, 1984.

Cranford, R. E., and Roberts, J. C. Biomedical ethics committees. *Primary Care* 13(2): 327–41, June 1986.

Greiner, G. G., and Storch, J. Hospital ethics committees: problems in evaluation. *HEC Forum* 4(1):5–18, 1992.

Middleton, C. Institutional ethics committees. *Ethics, Sponsorship, and Pastoral Ministry* 1(3):1–7, Summer 1992.

Miles, S. New business for ethics committees. *HEC Forum* 4(2):97–102, 1992.

Ross, J. W. *Handbook for Hospital Ethics Committees.* Chicago: American Hospital Publishing, 1986.

Seigler, M. Ethics committees: decisions by bureaucracy. *Hastings Center Report* 16(3):22–24, June 1986.

Euthanasia

Bok, S. Ethical views. Pt. II of death and dying, euthanasia and sustaining life: ethical views. In: W. T. Reich, editor. *Encyclopedia of Bioethics.* Vol. I. New York City: Free Press, 1978.

Graber, G., and Thomasma, D. *Euthanasia: Toward an Ethical Social Policy.* New York City: Continuum Press, 1990.

Horan, D., and Mall, D. *Death, Dying and Euthanasia.* Washington, DC: University Publications of America, 1977.

Kohl, M., editor. *Beneficent Euthanasia.* Buffalo, NY: Prometheus Books, 1975.

Meier, D. E. Physician assisted dying: theory and reality. *Journal of Clinical Ethics* 3(1):35–37, Spring 1992.

Rachels, J. *The End of Life: Euthanasia and Morality.* New York City: Oxford University Press, 1986.

Steinbock, B., editor. *Killing and Letting Die.* Englewood Cliffs, NJ: Prentice Hall, 1980.

Futility

Callahan, D. Medical futility: the problem without a name. *Hastings Center Report* 21(4):30–53, July–Aug. 1991.

Carter, B. S., and Sandling, J. Decision making in the NICU: the question of medical futility. *Journal of Clinical Ethics* 3(2):142–43, Summer 1992.

Coogan, M. Medical futility in resuscitation: value judgement and clinical judgement. *Cambridge Quarterly of Healthcare Ethics* (2):197–217, 1993.

Phillips, D., editor. Recent court decisions show wide range of rulings on futility. *Hospital Ethics* 7(6):1–4, Nov.–Dec. 1991.

Tomlinson, T., and Brody, H. Futility and the ethics of resuscitation. *JAMA* 264(10):1276–80, Sept. 12, 1990.

Nursing Ethics

Bandman, E. L., and Bandman, B. *Nursing Ethics through the Life Span.* 2nd ed. Norwalk, CT: Appleton and Lange, 1990.

Benjamin, M., and Curtis, J. *Ethics in Nursing.* 2nd ed. New York City: Oxford University Press, 1986.

Catalano, J. T., and Griffin, S. *Ethical and Legal Aspects of Nursing.* Springhouse, PA: Springhouse Corp., 1991.

Davis, A., and Aroskar, M. A. *Ethical Dilemmas and Nursing Practice.* 3rd ed. Norwalk, CT: Appleton and Lange, 1991.

Fairbairn, G., and Fairbairn, S., editors. *Ethical Issues in Caring.* Brookfield, VT: Avebury, 1988.

Melia, K. M. *Everyday Nursing Ethics.* Basingstoke, Hampshire, England: Macmillan Education, 1989.

Pence, T., and Cantrall, J. *Ethics in Nursing: An Anthology.* New York City: National League for Nursing, 1990.

Silva, M. C. *Ethical Decision Making in Nursing Administration.* Norwalk, CT: Appleton and Lange, 1990.

Thompson, I. E., Melia, K. M., and Boyde, K. M. *Nursing Ethics.* 2nd ed. New York City: Churchill Livingstone, 1988.

Veatch, R. M., and Fry, S. *Case Studies in Nursing Ethics.* Philadelphia: J. B. Lippincott, 1987.

Patient Self-Determination and Advance Directives

Brett, A. S. Limitations of listing specific medical interventions in advance directives. *JAMA* 266(6):825–28, Aug. 14, 1991.

Cole, H. M. Advance directives on admission: clinical implications and analysis of the Patient Self-Determination Act. *JAMA* 266(3):402–5, July 17, 1991.

Davis, M., Southerland, L. J., Garrett, J. M., Smith, J. L., Hielma, F., Pickard, G., Egner, D. M., and Patrick, D. L. A prospective study of advance directives for life-sustaining care. *New England Journal of Medicine* 324(13):882–87, Mar. 28, 1991.

Drane, J. F. The Patient Self-Determination Act (PSDA) and the incapacitated patient: policy suggestions for health care ethics committees. *HEC Forum* 3(6):309–20, 1991.

Faden, R., and Beauchamp, T. *History and Theory of Informed Consent.* New York City: Oxford University Press, 1986.

Mishkin, B. *A Matter of Choice: Planning Ahead for Health Care Decisions.* Washington, DC: American Association of Retired Persons, 1986.

Sehgal, A., Galbraith, A., Chesney, M., Schofield, P., Charles, G., and Lo, B. How strictly do dialysis patients want their advance directives followed? *JAMA* 267(1):59–63, Jan. 1, 1992.

Walton, D. *Physician-Patient Decision Making: A Study in Medical Ethics.* Westport, CT: Greenwood Press, 1985.

Winslade, W. J., and Ross, J. W. *Choosing Life or Death: A Guide for Patients, Families and Health Care Professionals.* New York City: Free Press, 1986.

Resuscitation

Bedel, S. E., and Delbanco, T. L. Choices about cardiopulmonary resuscitation in the hospital: when do physicians talk to patients? *New England Journal of Medicine* 310(17):1089–93, Apr. 26, 1984.

Emergency Cardiac Care Committee. Ethical considerations in resuscitation. *JAMA* 268(16):2282–88, Oct. 28, 1992.

Phillips, D. F., editor. New views define appropriate resuscitation circumstances. *Hospital Ethics* 8(1):1–5, Jan.–Feb. 1992.

Termination of Treatment/Life-Sustaining Treatment

Hackworth, C. B., editor. Discrimination law clashes with bioethics over PVS. *Medical Ethics Advisor* 7(7):81–96, July 1991.

Lynn, D. J. Deciding about life-sustaining treatment. In: C. K. Cassel and J. R. Walsh, editors. *Geriatric Medicine. Vol. II. Fundamentals of Geriatric Care.* New York City: Springer-Verlag, 1984.

Meisel, A. Legal myths about terminating life-support. *Archives of Internal Medicine* 151(8):1497–1502, Aug. 1991.

Murray, D., and Matcher, D. Life-sustaining therapy: a model for appropriate use. *JAMA* 264(16):1201–208, Oct. 24, 1990.

Neu, S., and Knellstrand, C. M. Stopping long term dialysis: an empirical study of withdrawal of life-supporting treatment. *New England Journal of Medicine* 314(1):14–20, June 2, 1986.

Phillips, D., editor. To treat or not to treat and who shall beg the question. *Hospital Ethics* 9(6):1–4, Dec. 1993.

Smith, D. H., and Veach, R., editors. *Guidelines on the Termination of Life-Sustaining Treatment and the Care of the Dying.* Bloomington, IN: Indiana University Press, 1987.

Task Force on Ethics of the Society of Critical Care Medicine. Consensus Report on the ethics of forgoing life-sustaining treatment in the critically ill. *Critical Care Medicine* 18(12):1435–39, Dec. 1990.

Toms, S. A. Outcome predictors in the early withdrawal of life-support: issues of justice and allocation for the severely brain injured. *Journal of Clinical Ethics* 4(3):206–11, Fall 1993.

Walton, D. N. *The Ethics of Withdrawal of Life-Supporting Systems: Case Studies on Decision Making in Intensive Care.* Westport, CT: Greenwood Press, 1983.

Weir, R. *Selective Non-Treatment of Handicapped Newborns: Moral Dilemmas in Neonatal Medicine.* New York City: Oxford University Press, 1984.

Weir, R., and Gostin, L. Decisions to abate life-sustaining treatment for non-autonomous patients. *JAMA* 264(14):1846–53, Oct. 10, 1990.

Videos

A Fate Worse than Death
This film discusses the issues related to whether to withdraw life support from a patient in a coma or in a persistent vegetative state. (50 minutes)
Fanlight Productions
47 Halifax St.
Boston, MA 02130
800/937-4113

A Matter of Life or Death
This program focuses on the bioethical dilemmas in the treatment of the terminally ill and questions whether it is wise to spend limited resources on individuals who are dying. (20 minutes)
Filmakers Library
124 East 40th St.
New York, NY 10016 212/808-4980

A Question of Ethics: The Dying Patient—Treating Pain
This film uses a hypothetical case to discuss issues of pain management and control, including the ethical issue of providing amounts of pain medication that have the potential to shorten a patient's life. (28 minutes)
AIMS Media
9710 DeSoto Ave.
Chattsworth, CA 91311-4409
800/367-2467

A Question of Ethics: A Heart Transplant Program
This video uses a hypothetical situation to explore the ethical aspects of a heart transplant program. (28 minutes)
AIMS Media
9710 DeSoto Ave.
Chattsworth, CA 91311-4409
800/367-2467

A Question of Ethics: Starting a Bio-Ethics Committee
This video on how to establish a bioethics committee includes information on the committee's function and roles of the individual members. (28 minutes)
AIMS Media
9710 DeSoto Ave.
Chattsworth, CA 91311-4409
800/367-2467

Born Dying
This film examines the plight of a family as they make treatment decisions for a dying newborn. (20 minutes)
Baxley Media Group
110 W. Main St.
Urbana, IL 61801-2700
217/384-4838

Caring for the Terminally Ill
This film emphasizes the goals of providing care and support to enhance the remaining time of terminally ill patients. It shows roles of family members and caregivers, and it reviews the emotional dimensions of this type of situation. (19 minutes)
Films for the Humanities and Sciences
P.O. Box 2053
Princeton, NJ 08543-2053
800/257-5126

Dax's Case
This film presents the case of a severely burned patient who requested to be allowed to die. His request was denied, and he lived. The film covers a 10-year span in which the patient continued to believe that he should have been allowed to die. (58 minutes)
Filmakers Library
124 East 40th St.
New York, NY 10016
212/808-4980

Decoding the Book of Life
This film provides information on the Human Genome Project. (58 minutes)
Films for the Humanities and Sciences
P.O. Box 2053
Princeton, NJ 08543-2053
800/257-5126

The DNR Dilemma
This is a two-part series. Part 1, *When the Time Comes*, dramatizes the issues faced by a physician who must discuss a do-not-resuscitate order with a patient. (18 minutes) Part 2, *Professional Perspectives*, provides commentary from health professionals who are affected by DNR orders. (25 minutes)
Baxley Media Group
110 W. Main St.
Urbana, IL 61801-2700
217/384-4838

Doctor Death: Medical Ethics and Doctor Assisted Suicide
This film offers an in-depth look at one physician's perspective on incurable illness and the ethical issues of doctor-assisted suicide. (28 minutes)
Films for the Humanities and Sciences
P.O. Box 2053
Princeton, NJ 08543-2053
800/257-5126

Dying Wish
This video discusses the decisions families have to make concerning termination of treatment or resuscitation of severely ill patients. (52 minutes)
Films for the Humanities and Sciences
P.O. Box 2053
Princeton, NJ 08543-2053
800/257-5126

Ethics Committees and the Handicapped Newborn
This film addresses the problems for both the hospital and family related to treatment decisions for infants born with severe birth defects. (30 minutes)
AIMS Media
9710 DeSoto Ave.
Chattsworth, CA 91311-4409
800/367-2467

Help Me Die
This program presents a discussion of the ethical issues that arise when a terminally ill patient asks a physician or a family member to provide assistance to end his or her life. (48 minutes)
Fanlight Productions
47 Halifax St.
Boston, MA 02130
800/937-4113

In the Middle of the End
This film provides a series of scenarios that can be used as a starting point in discussions about bioethical dilemmas. (29 minutes)
Center for Aging
College of Nursing/Pharmacy
1836 Lomas Blvd. NE
University of New Mexico
Albuquerque, NM 87131-6086
505/277-0860

Is This Life Worth Living?
This video is a documentary that explains the ethical issues related to sustaining the life of severely impaired patients. (30 minutes)
Filmakers Library
124 East 40th St.
New York, NY 10016
212/808-4980

Living Choices
This film provides answers to frequently asked questions concerning living wills, durable powers of attorney, and advance directives. (16 minutes)
Baxley Media Group
110 W. Main St.
Urbana, IL 61801-2700
217/384-4838

Living Wills
This program examines living wills and advance directives and is a guide for patients in making decisions concerning the use of ventilators, artificial food and hydration, and drugs. (30 minutes)
Films for the Humanities and Sciences
P.O. Box 2053
Princeton, NJ 08543-2053
800/257-5126

Medicine and Mercy
This film examines the interplay between technology, ethics, and the quality of life. (26 minutes)
Films for the Humanities and Sciences
P.O. Box 2053
Princeton, NJ 08543-2053
800/257-5126

No Heroic Measures
This video examines the question of when to terminate life support, including nasogastric feeding and hyperalimentation therapy, for elderly, incompetent patients. (23 minutes)
Baxley Media Group
110 W. Main St.
Urbana, IL 61801-2700
217/384-4838

The Right to Decide
This video explores issues related to a patient's hopes, fears, and goals in relation to end-of-life decisions and life-support therapies. The program also reviews information on the Patient Self-Determination Act. (43 minutes)
Fanlight Productions
47 Halifax St.
Boston, MA 02130
800/937-4113

The Right to Die
This film examines the legal, ethical, and emotional issues surrounding a patient's decision to have a ventilator turned off. (19 minutes)
Baxley Media Group
110 W. Main St.
Urbana, IL 61801-2700
217/384-4838

Who Lives—Who Dies?
This program examines the ethical issues concerning the rationing of health care and the provision of "useless" treatment to dying patients while others are in need of basic health care services. (58 minutes)
Filmakers Library
124 East 40th St.
New York, NY 10016
212/808-4980

Glossary

Advance directive: A format through which an adult can provide information about his or her desires concerning treatment choices in the event of future incapacity. An advance directive is usually in the form of a living will, a durable power of attorney for health care, or a directive to a physician. Although an advance directive is usually thought of as a written document, information concerning future treatment wishes can also be given verbally. Advance directives are invoked only if the patient is unable to act on his or her own behalf. Specifics concerning the legal aspects of advance directives vary from state to state.

Agent: An individual designated through a durable power of attorney to make health care decisions on behalf of a particular patient.

Allocation of resources: The process by which physicians, institutions, and public-policy makers determine how, where, when, and for whom limited funds are expended, to provide the greatest good to those in need of health care services.

Artificial nutrition and hydration: The provision of food and water through tubes or by other means to a patient who is unable to eat or swallow.

Autonomy: The right of a competent individual to make informed choices concerning medical treatment and care; the right to have control over one's personal destiny through self-determination.

Beneficence: The obligation to do that which is good.

Benefit versus burden: The identified possible positive outcomes of particular activities, procedures, or courses of treatment weighed against the possible problems, difficulties, or undesirable outcomes that the provision of these services might cause.

Bioethicist: An individual who has the training, knowledge, and skills to provide guidance and understanding in the application of ethical theory to health care; a person who can provide information about the moral implications of health care choices and decisions.

Biomedical ethics (bioethics): The application of ethical principles and reasoning in a medical or health care setting.

Biomedical ethics committee (institutional ethics committee/ethics committee): A group of individuals within a health care setting whose responsibilities are to develop and update policies, review cases, provide education, and oversee ongoing activities related to biomedical ethics.

Brain death: Permanent cessation of the functioning of all parts of the brain, including both hemispheres and the brain stem (as opposed to death as determined by the cessation of cardiovascular function).

CODE: The provision of cardiopulmonary resuscitation (CPR) or other life-saving measures to a patient in whom heart and lung function has ceased.

Coercion: The deliberate attempt to force an individual to act in a certain way or to make a particular decision.

Comfort measures: Procedures, treatments, and medicines provided to a terminally ill patient to keep that patient free from pain and discomfort. Comfort measures are not intended to effect a cure or an alteration in the disease process or to prolong life.

Competent versus incompetent: The ability versus the inability (as defined by a legal proceeding) to make or articulate wise, appropriate, logical choices concerning personal, medical, or financial matters.

Confidentiality: The professional, legal, and moral obligation not to obtain or divulge private information.

Decision-making capacity: The ability of an individual to receive, understand, and evaluate information and to make and communicate personal choices based on that information.

Deontology: The theory or study of moral obligation; the obligation not only to do things that produce good consequences but also to avoid doing things that would have unpleasant consequences.

Dignity: The respect and veneration shown to an individual that validates his or her worth, importance, and quality.

DNR (do not resuscitate) (no CODE): A decision (documented in the patient's chart) not to perform cardiopulmonary resuscitation in the event that the patient's heart and lung function ceases.

Durable power of attorney: A legal document that designates that a specific individual has the right to make health care decisions or other decisions on behalf of another individual. The durable power of attorney is activated only when a person becomes unable to make or articulate personal decisions.

Ethical decision making: The process that draws on ethical principles, theory, and precedents to make judgments, choices, and decisions.

Ethical dilemma: A situation in which a conflict of moral values or beliefs results in differences of opinion concerning treatment or care options for a particular patient or group of individuals.

Ethics: A philosophical discipline defined as the study of good and evil, right and wrong, and duty and obligation in human contact.

Ethics consult: A formal procedure that provides a forum (usually through an ethics committee) for physicians, nurses, and other identified health care workers to address questions and concerns about the ethical implications of care and treatment for a specific patient.

Euthanasia: An action (active euthanasia) or omission (passive euthanasia) that intentionally causes death. Also known as *mercy killing*, euthanasia is intended to end the perceived suffering of a patient.

Futility: The belief or conclusion that a particular medical treatment or therapy would be of no benefit to a patient and that it should not be prescribed or carried out.

Genetic engineering: The scientific alteration or manipulation of DNA in a gene, with the goal of eliminating or treating a genetic disorder or creating a change within an organism.

Guardian (legal): A person who is appointed through a court proceeding to care for another (incompetent) individual and to make personal, medical, or financial decisions on that person's behalf (as opposed to an agent, who is selected by the patient and designated through a durable power of attorney to make health care decisions only).

Informed consent: The legal and moral requirement that a physician must obtain permission to perform any medical procedure. The permission must be obtained from the patient if he or she is competent or from a surrogate decision maker if the patient is incompetent. Before obtaining permission, the physician is obligated to provide all relevant and complete information concerning risks, benefits, alternatives, and possible outcomes of the procedure being recommended.

Justice: Equitable and reasonable distribution of care, goods, and services.

Life-sustaining treatment (life support): A medical procedure using mechanical and artificial methods of maintaining or restoring a vital function. When used with a terminally ill patient, life support serves to artificially maintain bodily function and to postpone the moment of death. (Life-support equipment is used to artificially maintain organ systems in brain-dead patients whose organs are to be harvested, or obtained, for transplantation.)

Living will: A written, signed form of an advance directive that describes (often in great detail) what forms of life-sustaining treatments an individual would or would not want in the event of a future catastrophic event or illness. A living will enables the physician and other caregivers to have guidance and information about treatment choices, which the patient is not able to communicate directly at the time that the living will is invoked. Specific laws and requirements about living wills vary from state to state. Because there is no single correct way to write a living will, details of the design and the specifications within the document will differ from person to person.

Nonmaleficence: Exercising care to do no harm.

Ordinary versus extraordinary care: Medical treatment or procedures that are standard for the time, place, and situation versus treatment or procedures that are considered heroic or futile or that exceed the norm; also can be referred to as proportionate versus disproportionate care.

Organ and tissue donation: An arrangement whereby usable body parts are harvested (obtained) from a deceased patient and transplanted into a living individual.

Persistent vegetative state (PVS): A relatively stable neurological condition characterized by wakefulness without awareness of self or environment. Individuals in a PVS are alive but are incapable of intellectual or social interaction.

Philosophical grounding: A belief system that is based on logic, reason, judgment, and systematic analysis.

Physician-assisted suicide: A course of action through which a terminally or chronically ill patient intentionally causes his or her own death, with the full advance knowledge of a physician, who may or may not be present at the time of the death. The patient dies as a result of following instructions provided by the physician, through the administration of drugs prescribed by the physician, or through a specific act performed by either the physician or another individual.

Quality of life: The degree to which an individual's existence is perceived worthwhile based on a combination of subjective factors.

Significant other: The individual who is emotionally closest to a patient and who is most likely to be aware of the patient's wishes and to have the patient's best interests at heart.

Slippery slope: A colloquial term describing the phenomena that result when one course of action leads to another, and yet another, causing ultimate changes and consequences that may not have been intended or wanted. For example, in the 1970s and 1980s, situations concerning inappropriate treatment of a few institutionalized mentally ill and mentally retarded patients were brought before the courts. This led to a review of all such facilities and many mental health institutions to "protect" the civil rights of the patients. This review resulted in the discharge of many marginally capable individuals who had no place to go. Some of these patients were subsequently placed in group homes or in semi-independent living situations, from which they later were allowed to leave. The result has been that many former patients remain ill and are now street people with little or no meaningful support or assistance.

Social-cultural grounding: A belief system that is based on heritage, ancestry, nationality, family background, and community values.

Surrogate (proxy) decision maker: A person who makes health care and end-of-life choices on behalf of another individual. In some cases, a surrogate is legally appointed to serve in this capacity. In other cases, a significant other may assume the role.

Terminal condition: An incurable, irreversible state caused by illness or injury.

Termination of treatment: The conscious decision to forgo additional medical procedures.

Theological grounding: A belief system based on faith, religious heritage, or the values expressed in a specific religion, sect, or denomination.

Treatment decision: A choice concerning the provision of a specific type of medical care.

Utilitarianism: A theory that the purpose and aim of actions should be to obtain the best possible ratio of pleasure to pain or the greatest happiness for the greatest number of people.

Values: Deeply held cultural and personal beliefs that drive human behavior. Values are laden with an emotional charge in that they provide the framework for the *shoulds* and the *should nots* that define and protect an individual, a group, or a culture. They are often articulated in religious statements (for example, the Ten Commandments) or political documents (the Bill of Rights). Values often create powerful, nonnegotiable standards by which people live.

Veracity: The devotion or obligation to be honest and to provide all facts and information without bias, interpretation, misrepresentation, or misguidance.

Withdrawal of treatment: The removal of a patient from an existing level of care.

Withholding of treatment: The decision not to begin a particular level of care.

Appendix

The Noncompliant Patient: A Biomedical Ethics Grand Rounds Program

The following discussion is a fictionalized adaptation and brief synopsis of an actual grand rounds program. Although the basic concept and flow of the program remain intact, all patient and staff information and names have been changed to protect confidentiality. Any resemblance to actual persons is entirely coincidental.

Educator: Good afternoon. I'm Dr. Campbell from the hospital's educational services department, and I'd like to welcome you to our biomedical ethics grand rounds program. In our discussion today, we will focus on the ethical issues surrounding the noncompliant patient—that individual who, for one reason or another, does not follow recommendations, ends up back in the hospital, and generally causes difficulty for the staff on many levels.

Our panel today consists of Ms. Jones, a nurse on our dialysis unit; Mrs. Gordon, a home health nurse; and Dr. Thomas, one of the psychologists on our physical medicine and rehabilitation unit. Each of the panel members will give a brief synopsis of the case of a noncompliant patient for whom there have been ethical issues and concerns. Following these presentations, Dr. Smith, our hospital ethicist, will lead a discussion concerning the ethical dimensions of the cases.

Ms. Jones: The case that I am going to present is that of Miss A. She has been a patient in the dialysis unit for four years. She is in her late 50s and is very noncompliant. This patient has diabetes, and her blood sugar level ranges from very high to very low. Many times she does not show up for a treatment as prescribed, and then we have to contact the police to go to her home to check on her. When the police get there, they often find her unconscious, and they then call the paramedics to bring her to the emergency department.

This patient refuses to follow the treatment that was prescribed. She doesn't lose the weight she is supposed to, she doesn't try to stabilize her blood sugar, and so forth.

Miss A. usually comes here in the hospital's van, but we've had a lot of problems with her not being ready when the van arrives or with her refusing to open the door. When she doesn't use the van, she is supposed to make her own transportation arrangements with a taxi, but she can't afford it, so she just doesn't show up. When that happens, we send the police.

At one point, Miss A. did drive. We felt that she was very unsafe behind the wheel, so with the help of her physician we had her license revoked. That caused a lot of problems, too. She was very angry with us, but we were convinced that for her own safety, it was the right thing to do.

In the past month, Miss A. was admitted to our intensive care unit after she had a heart attack. She signed herself out—AMA. We then had the problem of her refusal to follow our treatment recommendations concerning not only dialysis and diabetes but also her heart condition.

The question that we have is, Where do our responsibilities begin and end? We are an outpatient dialysis center, so do our responsibilities start and stop when the patient walks through the door, or do we need to follow the patients when they get home? Are we supposed to ensure that they are following the recommended treatments? When they don't show up, should we really be contacting the police?

Mrs. Gordon: Mr. B. is a 66-year-old patient who has multiple sclerosis. He became our patient in 1990 and received physical and occupational therapy in his home. At that time, he was able to use a quad cane to get around. He was also able to prepare his own meals and provide for his own self-care needs. A year later, his ability to care for himself began to decline. He could no longer cook, and his personal hygiene was very poor. Friends brought meals and helped with some of his basic needs, but he was essentially trying to make do.

Mr. B. was no longer able to walk at all and got around in an electric cart. During the next three years, he had ups and downs in his ability to care for himself but was generally unable to provide for most of his basic needs. He had frequent admissions to the rehabilitation unit of the hospital for treatment after falls. The last time he was discharged from rehab, the staff expressed serious concerns that he was no longer able to live at home.

The patient, however, was certain that he could still live independently and insisted on returning to his home. He stated that he would be safer there and that he didn't want any changes in his lifestyle.

Mr. B. was no longer able to transfer independently to the toilet and refused to have a commode in the bedroom. He was incontinent of both stool and urine and would often remain in the same diaper from early morning until late evening. He developed severe decubitus ulcers.

The patient had a portable phone but frequently forgot to keep it with him. As a result, when he fell, which was often, he frequently was not found for several hours. Recently, Mr. B. did have his phone with him when he fell, and he called 911. He was not injured, so the police called our home health department to ask what we were going to do about the patient.

Mr. B. is now being seen by home health nurses on a daily basis. However, he is alone for most of the rest of the day. Our staff believes that he should be admitted to a nursing home, but the patient has refused. Home health staff are concerned for this patient's health, safety, and welfare and are frustrated because his living condition makes successful treatment almost impossible.

Dr. Thomas: Mrs. C. is a 51-year-old married woman who has a college education. She was admitted to our physical medicine and rehabilitation unit five months ago after suffering a stroke on the right side of her brain, which affected the left side of her body.

This patient worked with her husband at a bookstore on weekends and on some weekdays. She seemed to be generally happy with her life, and when she was first admitted, she appeared to be open and friendly. She was forthcoming with information and seemed to have an understanding of what was facing her.

The more I spoke with her, however, the more it became apparent that she was easily agitated and somewhat depressed. When I shared this observation with her, she stated that she had always been that way.

Mrs. C. also told me that she was a heavy smoker and drank several bottles of wine a week. I don't know if that information is relevant, but I think it's an important element of her personality.

Mrs. C. was able to state that she was depressed over the fact that she had suffered a stroke. With time, she became more and more agitated, and that agitation seemed to be directed toward her husband. As we discussed these issues, she admitted that perhaps she could use some supportive therapy. She was referred to our stroke support group, and she agreed to go. At first it appeared that she intended to go along with her therapy program.

Soon after that, I was called to the patient's room because she had decided to go home. She stated that she had "business to take care of" and that she was leaving. She was unyielding and inflexible. Her husband grudgingly went along with everything she said.

I attempted to explain that she would not have the support at home that she needed and that she was still in need of physical therapy. Although she seemed to listen, it was clear that she did not fully understand the implications of this choice. She had made up her mind that she was going home, and I felt that she was kind of bullying her husband to agree. The patient subsequently signed herself out of the unit.

About six weeks later, Mrs. C. was readmitted to the unit. She was still suffering the aftereffects of the stroke, of course, but in addition—because she had not kept up with her physical therapy—she had an occlusion in the artery in her left leg, which necessitated a below-the-knee amputation. The patient was now in worse shape than she had been in when we first saw her. When I spoke to her later, she did admit to having some responsibility for what had happened to her, but she was also very angry to be back in the hospital.

Mrs. C. was not nearly as friendly or as personable as she had been when I first saw her. It soon became apparent that she again did not want to stay in the hospital and that she wanted to go home. Her ability to relate to others was poor, and she was more depressed than she had been before. Mrs. C. stated that she had thoughts of suicide and even admitted that she had a supply of sleeping pills hidden at home. She told me where they were and allowed me to call her husband so that he could dispose of them.

Mrs. C. did stay on the unit and reluctantly received therapy, but she frequently threatened to leave, and we were never sure just what she would do. It was difficult for the staff to work with her.

Dr. Smith (ethicist): We have heard the cases. Part of ethics, when you are trying to look at ethical dilemmas, is to ask the question, What is it about these situations that causes us to have a dilemma? In other words, what are the problems that occurred in these particular cases?

First of all, do you have any questions to ask the presenters about these cases? Do you need more clarification or information that will help you understand the cases better as we look for a solution?

Audience member (nurse): I'm wondering if anybody talked to these patients besides the treating person. In all three cases, there is obviously the appearance of irresponsibility on the part of the patient, but I wonder if there isn't also an inherent fear of the hospital environment in which these people found themselves. Did these patients have a fear of losing control or being imprisoned in the sterile environment? Was that what they were running away from?

Audience member (home health nurse A): We had a social worker visit Mr. B. to see if we could help him make some sort of a plan—something that would put him in a safer environment. The social worker was someone he hadn't met while he was in the hospital. It was the home health social worker. But he was firm in his decision to stay in his home because it was *his* home.

Dr. Smith: He was secure there?

Audience member (home health nurse A): Right.

Dr. Smith: Does anybody have any other questions? . . . Then let me ask you this. In all three cases, what *is* the ethical issue?

Audience member (chaplain): What about patient autonomy?

Dr. Smith: What *about* patient autonomy—the right of patients to ask for help when they need it and the responsibility of the health care providers to try to provide what patients want. If we really believe in autonomy, once we give them autonomy and they are on their own, why is their outcome our problem? . . . Right?

Audience member (chaplain): I think he has a point.

Dr. Smith: So, do we really even have an ethical issue here?

Audience member (social worker A): We often see patients who, in our opinion, are endangering their lives because of their actions and the choices they are making. We believe that we should offer something to them that would help things be different if they cooperated with us. But then autonomy is an issue . . .

Dr. Smith: If they don't want what you are offering, aren't you forcing something on them? Is that a violation of their autonomy? Their dignity?

Audience member (social worker A): I guess it depends on a lot of things. In the case presented by Dr. Thomas, there might have been a discussion that we in social work could have helped in this case. Maybe we could have helped the patient with the understanding of her situation. Then the decision to leave the hospital prematurely might have changed.

Dr. Thomas: The first time she was in the hospital, she didn't give us a chance to get you involved.

I guess another aspect of the autonomy issue is that patients not only put their own lives in jeopardy but they also cause problems for other people. The first time Mrs. C. left the hospital against medical advice, it was explained to her that her husband wasn't trained as a physical therapist and that if he attempted to do things like transfer her or move her, they both could get hurt.

Audience member (social worker B): I think another thing to point out in the autonomy issue is that in our state the law comes down heavily on the side of patient autonomy. It is very difficult for anyone to get guardianship. It's hard to get, especially if the patient is mentally oriented, no matter what kinds of decisions the patient is making. Guardianship might be a possibility under extreme cases, but there will be a legal-aid attorney appointed to be on the side of autonomy—so it's hard.

Audience member (home health nurse A): From a home care standpoint, we did not feel that Mr. B. was mentally competent to be making the decisions he was making, and yet we were told by his doctors that he was. So, we had an ethical problem because we really did not feel he was capable of making these decisions.

Dr. Smith: I'm going to challenge you on that one. You said you felt that he was not competent. Can you give us an indication of why you felt that way? I'm looking for more than just an opinion here. Do you have some specific information in this area?

Audience member (home health nurse A): This man had multiple sclerosis, and from the time we opened a file on him, he had severe short-term memory loss. We could not tell him anything without him writing everything down on notes. He had piles and piles of notes all over his home. But then he would forget where he put the note he wanted and couldn't remember what he had written down.

Dr. Smith: He probably knew himself that he could not remember things for very long.

Audience member (home health nurse A): But he thought he was in control simply because he was writing things down.

Dr. Thomas: Mr. B. is a patient whom we had also seen on the rehab unit. We also had concerns about his going home, especially if he was going home alone, but we learned that he intended to take in boarders to help out, so we were under the impression that he would be taken care of. It was clear, however, that he did not have a complete understanding of his own deficits.

Audience member (home health nurse B): On the first home visit we learned that the boarders—who were new—were not going to be involved in Mr. B.'s care. Mr. B. was incontinent, and the boarders didn't want anything to do with his personal care. They would help cook and clean, but that was all. They also didn't want to get involved in Mr. B.'s safety. Once, when he fell, they called the doctor and got very angry because Mr. B. couldn't pick himself up. They didn't think he should have been sent home. They didn't want to be responsible for him.

Also, Mr. B. was afraid of the boarders. There was a lot of discussion and whispering when they were around, and he was even afraid to go into their room, which is where the phone is kept. That was why sometimes he had the phone with him and sometimes he didn't, even though he was instructed to keep it near him.

When we called both physicians who were his primary care providers, they told us that they had promised not to place him into a long-term care facility until he was ready to go. The doctors stated to me that they thought that Mr. B. was competent to make this decision, even though I told them that I had every health care discipline in there.

Dr. Smith: Let me ask you this. Do you think it was fair to promise him that he would not be placed in a facility unless he was ready? None of us know everything there is to know when we make most decisions. And now people are trying to keep a promise that maybe shouldn't have been made in the first place.

Audience member (home health nurse B): That's right.

Audience member (physical therapist): There's one point that I'd like to make from a rehab perspective: we had a hard time convincing Mr. B. that when he was unable to do things in the hospital, he was still going to be unable to do them at home. When we went out to the home and assessed him using an electric cart before he was actually discharged, we didn't feel comfortable at all about his safety. When he did eventually go home, home health nurses found the same thing—that he couldn't use the cart and that he wasn't safe. Since then, he's had 10 or 11 admissions back on the rehab unit. This just keeps going on and on. Where do you draw the line?

Dr. Smith: That's a good question.

Audience member (social worker C): I was involved with Mr. B. when he was on the rehab unit and through all of his many admissions, and safety at home after discharge was a constant issue for the team. It was discussed in detail, but despite everybody on the team trying to point out the safety risks, Mr. B. plainly said to us time and time again that *he* would decide when to leave his home. Also, we had no backup from the physicians, and the patient really trusted them.

Dr. Smith: So ultimately, what's the bottom line here? Who is responsible for this patient? Home health? The physician? Or the patient himself? The same thing is true for our other two cases. Doesn't the patient receiving dialysis have the right not to show up for treatment? And doesn't the stroke patient have the right to leave the hospital?

I'm reminded of the story of a family I knew not too long ago. They were struggling with the issue of placing the mother in a nursing home. The father was feeling very guilty, and I remember the daughter saying, "Dad, Mom had lots of choices to make in her life. She never decided to choose things that would lead to good health. Her diet was poor. She didn't exercise. She did whatever she wanted to do. Those choices put her in her present condition. We've got to get on with the rest of our lives. We can't take responsibility for her choices."

What's your reaction to that story? Is this point of view right or wrong?

Audience member (social worker A): Well, sometimes that is not so easy to live with. We can say, "Well, OK, it's the patient's choice—what can we do?" But I find that often that kind of thinking doesn't satisfy me. You have to go a little further. I just have trouble with it.

Dr. Smith: Does anyone have a different perspective?

Audience member (community guest): Nobody consciously wants to bring harm to themselves. If a person makes a choice that is not in his or her best interest, don't health care workers sometimes have a better perspective? Can't the patients be told that they aren't making the right choices? Isn't there an obligation to correct faulty reasoning?

Dr. Smith: Another good question.

Audience member (chaplain): Who is going to draw that line? Who is going to decide what's faulty? Who is to determine that this is a time we can make the better choice or that this time it's still OK for the patient to make the choice?

Dr. Smith: Here you have several patients. You want to respect their integrity and autonomy as far as they are being exercised *appropriately*—and that's a big word here. You also have physicians who are the primary decision makers for these patients, and you need to remember that they are the only ones who practice medicine. The hospital staff does not practice medicine; they are there to support the physicians. When physicians and staff don't agree, conflict and confusion result. But somebody has to make a decision.

Audience member (volunteer): The health professionals have to point out what is in the patient's best interest. They have to say, "In my opinion, this would be the best choice for you." But in the final analysis, the patient should have the autonomy to say, "No, this is the way I'm going to do it." That doesn't present any ethical problem.

Dr. Smith: Even if the patient writes things down and then forgets where he put them? Even if the patient doesn't get dialysis and might die? Even if we end up having to amputate someone's leg because she left the hospital and didn't get proper care?

Audience member (volunteer): If a patient *is* incompetent, then it should be brought to the physician's attention, and he or she should take the proper steps. Then we can step in.

Audience member (home health nurse B): The second question is, Do we continue to care for these patients? Do we keep spending resources for dialysis patients who don't comply? Does home health continue to see patients like Mr. B. when we're really not meeting his needs?

Dr. Smith: That is exactly the issue. With Mr. B. we have a patient who would rather live in a compromised state, reaching out for whatever freedom is left, rather than make the choice to leave home.

In the professionals' opinions, we don't really have enough evidence to say that Mr. B. is incompetent. So he stays home. We're respecting his autonomy when we let him live that way, and maybe there is nothing we can do about it. But should we provide care for him now? He's going to end up being brought back into the hospital. Should we say that this is a waste of money?

Are we, in a sense, punishing him for making what we feel is a wrong choice? . . . If he doesn't agree with us, then we won't provide care?

Or should we just say that the best we can do is support him in his autonomy and be there for him if he needs us?

Audience member (physician): There are laws to protect incompetent people from themselves. Unfortunately, there are no laws against bad judgment. Certainly we can't permit ourselves to deny care simply on the basis of a prior episode of poor judgment.

A lot of people wouldn't get any medical care if we did that. It would be unethical to deny care simply on the basis of how a person chose to live.

Mrs. Gordon: Home care has a slightly different problem because home care is sent out to visit the patient for one hour per day. During that one hour we can give service, but when we are not there, patients are often on their own.

Therefore, in cases like Mr. B.'s, the service we can provide is not adequate. It's not service we are proud of, because it is not enough.

When we give the patient one hour of service, are we enabling the patient to stay in an unsafe environment? He or she will then think, "I can stay here because a nurse will be here tomorrow." If we didn't give that care, would it force the patient to make a different decision?

Dr. Smith: Is a little care worse than no care at all? Maybe, like an alcoholic, this patient would bottom out and realize that without any help, he'd die in that situation. But is that the kind of thing we want to impose on somebody?

Mrs. Gordon: When we can't meet our standard, we feel totally inadequate. Don't we have the right to give the care that we know is correct?

Dr. Smith: There is a conflict of rights here. But let me ask you this: Whose rights predominate here? Everybody is challenged. We have the right as professionals to practice professionally according to set standards, and here are people in need of serious help, but we can't practice according to those standards. What should we do?

Audience member (physician): You swallow your pride and do it, or you find someone else who will.

Audience member (nurse): It sounds as if we're being put in a position to have to evaluate how someone chooses to live or die. From our perspective it may not be a meaningful choice, but if it's meaningful to them, then it's OK. We can't go in with our own values about how they are going to spend the rest of their lives.

We can't refuse to take care of people because of their choices. If we did that, we wouldn't treat all the diabetics, heart patients, and addicts who come here.

But another thing we really have to be aware of is how the patient's choices affect other people in their lives. If they are making choices that have an impact on others, then maybe we do have to step in.

Dr. Smith: That's a good distinction to make.

Audience member (volunteer): In relation to Mr. B., I have a question as to why the physician didn't understand the reality of what was going on. When the patient fell and the police called us, why weren't they told to call the physician instead?

Audience member (home health nurse B): We did that once. The physician's solution was to tell the police to call the paramedics, and the patient was brought to the emergency department and admitted. The physician never got to the patient's home to see the situation there.

Dr. Smith: So there is really a communication problem here, isn't there? Where is the forum for addressing these problems? Where can you gather all the people who are interested in a particular case to sit down and present all the issues and come to some kind of a consensus?

In so many cases—not just home care—there are many health care disciplines involved, and no one but the family is aware of everything that is going on. If there is no coordination among disciplines, that in itself is an ethical issue.

And these cases raise another interesting issue. It's relatively easy to deal with patients who are competent, and we're clear on what to do for patients who are incompetent, but these three patients seem to fall through the cracks, and we care for a lot of people like them. They are not incompetent, but they seem to be making poor judgments. What should we do?

Audience member (social worker): If we have a patient who is alert and oriented but making poor judgments, frequently there will be a loving relative who will step in and work with us to help the patient. That usually works out very well. The problem comes in cases such as these when there isn't anyone else. That's when we need more help.

Dr. Smith: Is help available?

Audience member (nurse): Through an ethics committee consult?

Dr. Smith: Exactly. Any member of any of the teams of professionals who work with patients can contact the ethics committee and ask for a consult. The ethics committee would then gather the interested parties together, so that all of the issues could be put on the table and discussed. It's a way to open communication and a way to give everyone a chance to be in the same place at the same time so that the issues can be looked at logically.

Our time, unfortunately, is up for now. Of course, we are left with many questions and more food for thought, but I would like to reinforce one final point before we adjourn. We must remember that competent patients *do* have the right to refuse treatment. We can make recommendations and suggestions, but we must respect patients' autonomy and allow them to make their own informed choices.